Neuropsychology for Occupational Therapists

Neuropsychology for Occupational Therapists

Cognition in Occupational Performance

Fourth Edition

Edited by

Linda Maskill
College of Health and Life Sciences,
Brunel University London, UK

Stephanie Tempest
College of Occupational Therapists, London, UK

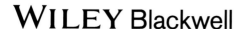
WILEY Blackwell

Registered Offices
John Wiley & Sons, Inc., 111 River Street, Hoboken, NJ 07030, USA
John Wiley & Sons Ltd, The Atrium, Southern Gate, Chichester, West Sussex, PO19 8SQ, UK

Editorial Office
9600 Garsington Road, Oxford, OX4 2DQ, UK

For details of our global editorial offices, customer services, and more information about Wiley products visit us at www.wiley.com.

Wiley also publishes its books in a variety of electronic formats and by print-on-demand. Some content that appears in standard print versions of this book may not be available in other formats.

Library of Congress Cataloging-in-Publication Data

Names: Maskill, Linda, 1959– editor. | Tempest, Stephanie, 1975– editor. | Preceded by (work): Grieve, June I. Neuropsychology for occupational therapists.
Title: Neuropsychology for occupational therapists : cognition in occupational performance / edited by Linda Maskill, Stephanie Tempest.
Description: Fourth edition. | Hoboken, NJ : John Wiley & Sons Inc., [2017] | Preceded by Neuropsychology for occupational therapists / June Grieve, Linda Gnanasekaran. 3rd ed. 2008. | Includes bibliographical references and index.
Identifiers: LCCN 2016053374 | ISBN 9781118711323 (pbk.) | ISBN 9781118711316 (Adobe PDF) | ISBN 9781118711309 (ePub)
Subjects: | MESH: Neuropsychology–methods | Occupational Therapy–methods | Neurocognitive Disorders–diagnosis | Perception–physiology | Memory Disorders–diagnosis | Motor Skills Disorders–diagnosis | Neurologic Examination
Classification: LCC RC386.6.N48 | NLM WL 103.5 | DDC 616.8/0475–dc23
LC record available at https://lccn.loc.gov/2016053374

Cover image: Science Photo Library – PASIEKA/Gettyimages

Set in 10/12pt Warnock by SPi Global, Pondicherry, India
Printed and bound in Malaysia by Vivar Printing Sdn Bhd

10 9 8 7 6 5 4 3 2

Contents

About the Editors

Linda Maskill MSc BSc(Hons) DipCOT FHEA

Linda has worked in higher education for 27 years, teaching student occupational therapists and physiotherapists at undergraduate and postgraduate levels. She is a senior lecturer in occupational therapy and the Departmental Director for Learning and Teaching, in the Department of Clinical Sciences at Brunel University London. Her teaching and scholarship focus upon physiology, neurology, ageing, cognition and neurorehabilitation. She has a particular interest in ageing and frailty. Prior to teaching, Linda worked in neurorehabilitation and community physical disability services.

Stephanie Tempest PhD MSc PGCert LTHE BSc(Hons) FHEA

Stephanie is the Education Manager for Professional Development at the College of Occupational Therapists (COT). Prior to this, she worked at Brunel University London, teaching occupational therapy and neurorehabilitation students at undergraduate and postgraduate levels. She has a clinical background in neurosciences and stroke rehabilitation. Stephanie has published a number of articles in peer-reviewed journals and contributed to the third edition of this text. She was a reviewer for the fifth edition of the National Clinical Guidelines for Stroke. Her research interests are varied and include the *International Classification of Functioning, Disability and Health* (ICF), service development, cognition and the lived experience of disability. A central theme throughout her career is supporting lifelong learning for the benefit of those who use services.

About the Contributors

Tess Baird MSc Bsc(Hons)

Tess graduated as an occupational therapist from Oxford Brookes University in 1995. She has worked in the field of neurology, specifically stroke, for over 20 years. Tess completed her MSc Neurorehabilitation at Brunel University London in 2005, publishing the output from her dissertation. She has worked across London in hyperacute, inpatient and community neurology and stroke teams. She has been actively involved with the College of Occupational Therapists – Specialist Section in Neurological Practice including the London Committee and the National Committee, via the Stroke Forum. She was part of the team collaborating on the recent COT/ACPIN Clinical Guidelines for splinting. Tess is currently the Clinical Lead for Stroke in Barts Health, managing therapists working across hyperacute, acute and community stroke rehabilitation, and is part of the training staff for 'Bridges – Self Management in Stroke'.

Sacha Hildebrandt MSc BSc

Sacha qualified at the University of Cape Town, South Africa, in 2000 and spent her first seven years working in London NHS hospitals specialising in adult neurorehabilitation. Since returning to South Africa, she has worked in private healthcare in Johannesburg and is the Clinical Director of Occupational Therapy in a multidisciplinary neurorehabilitation practice. Sacha's areas of particular interest include cognitive rehabilitation, vocational rehabilitation and return to driving.

Richard Jefferson MSc PGCE DipCOT

Richard has worked primarily in neurology since graduating from the London School of Occupational Therapy in 1988. He gained his MSc Neurorehabilitation from Brunel University London in 1999 and completed a Postgraduate Certificate in Education at Greenwich University in 2006. His career has moved from acute inpatient to community neurorehabilitation and developing clinical services with the brain injury charity Headway. Previous positions have included clinical lead and specialist posts in community neurology teams. Currently Richard is writing up his PhD thesis exploring the introduction of the *International Classification of Functioning, Disability and Health* (ICF) into clinical practice. He has published on this subject and presented nationally and internationally on both the introduction of the ICF and neurorehabilitation. When not working in neurology, he taught rehabilitation in Malawi and worked as a community therapist in Canada.

Preface

This book was written primarily for pre-registration students and novice practitioners of occupational therapy. Experienced practitioners will find a useful review of frameworks used within the profession to structure assessment and intervention, together with an update of knowledge in neuropsychology. Members of the multidisciplinary team will gain an insight into the unique role of the occupational therapist in cognitive rehabilitation.

The first edition of *Neuropsychology for Occupational Therapists* was written at a time when cognitive rehabilitation was becoming one of the major areas of occupational therapy practice. The aim was to create an understanding of the part played by cognition, and the effects of its impairment, in daily living.

Relevant assessments of perception and cognition were presented and developed further in the second edition to reflect an increase in the number of standardised assessments available. In the third edition, Linda Gnanasekaran (now Maskill) introduced chapters that related the study of cognitive functions and impairment to current occupational therapy practice. In this fourth edition, Linda Maskill has been joined by Stephanie Tempest to further update the content and introduce new material relating to the maintenance of cognitive health and function in later years. Guest contributors, occupational therapists and experts in their fields of practice, have updated the chapters on attention, memory and executive functions.

Part 1 introduces cognition within the context of occupational performance, emphasising its pivotal role. An occupational focus for cognitive rehabilitation is proposed based upon two theoretical frameworks: one an internationally recognised framework and classification for health and health-related states, the other specific to occupational therapy. The value of these frameworks is explored in relation to the occupational therapy process, exemplifying how theoretical constructs, core skills and knowledge are combined to achieve a rigorous approach to rehabilitation. Not only the student or novice practitioner but also experienced practitioners are given a succinct review of the occupational therapy process. Part 1 establishes the therapeutic context for the knowledge presented in Part 2.

Part 2 outlines the theoretical background for each of the components of the cognitive system and describes the disorders associated with their impairment. The presentation of cognitive functions in separate chapters facilitates both the discussion of relevant research in neuropsychology and the presentation of detailed knowledge. It must, however, be remembered that occupational therapists are often confronted with people who present with multiple impairments. The challenges of ageing and maintaining healthy cognitive function are addressed in a new chapter (11), that reflects current concerns about multimorbidity and cognitive impairments in later years. Activities in earlier editions, that encourage the reader to focus on their own cognitive abilities, have been retained and extended. Case studies have been retained, and summaries of the functional consequences of disorders reinforce the effects of impairment on function. Narratives of the lived experience have been included for the first time, to further illustrate the impact of cognitive impairments upon occupational performance.

Part 2 carries over the general guidelines given in Part 1 to suggestions for assessment and intervention related to specific areas of cognition.

Our task of integrating basic knowledge with occupational therapy has proved daunting and exciting. If this text is found useful as a resource for neuropsychology, and for guidance to practice, then we have continued to uphold and build upon this aim as first expressed by June Grieve, its original author.

Linda and Stephanie

Acknowledgements

We owe an enormous debt of gratitude to June Grieve, the original author of *Neuropsychology for Occupational Therapists*, whose work made this fourth edition possible. June was an inspirational teacher and mentor, and we both had the honour and privilege of working with her on the third edition. We hope we have carried her spirit with us into this new edition. We also wish to acknowledge Jo Creighton, who produced original line drawings for all the preceding editions of this book, some of which appear again in this edition.

Our Thanks

We would like to express our thanks to Richard Jefferson, Tess Baird and Sacha Hildebrandt, who updated and revised Chapters 5, 8 and 10 respectively.

About the Companion Website

Don't forget to visit the companion website for this book:

www.wiley.com/go/maskill/neuropsychologyOT

There you will find valuable material designed to enhance your learning, including:
- interactive multiple choice questions
- links to further reading.

Part I

Cognition and the Occupational Therapy Process

Occupation and Cognitive Rehabilitation

Stephanie Tempest and Linda Maskill

AIMS

1) To understand cognition and the role of cognitive skills in occupational performance.
2) To introduce and discuss the importance of using two specific frameworks – the International Classification of Functioning, Disability and Health (ICF) and the Occupational Therapy Practice Framework (OTPF).
3) To demonstrate the use of the ICF and the OTPF to guide our analysis of occupational performance in cognitive rehabilitation.

What is Cognition?

Cognition is 'the process of obtaining knowledge through thought, experience and the senses' (*Oxford English Dictionary* 2005). It derives from a Latin verb, the meanings of which include to get to learn, to recognise and to find out.

Cognition is studied in many different disciplines and the meaning varies when applied to psychology, philosophy, linguistics or computer science. For example, in computer science, cognition includes the development of artificial intelligence and robotics.

But our understanding of cognition draws upon health science, neuropsychology and the concept of occupational performance. As therapists, we need to understand how the brain functions and subsequently dysfunctions following neurological insult, in specific cognitive modalities such as attention, memory and purposeful movement. Then we need to apply this knowledge of cognitive body functions to understand how people use them to build skills and to perform activities within the context of their everyday life.

There are different ways to classify cognitive functions and some of these debates will be evident in Part 2 when we seek definitions of 'individual' impairments. For the purposes of this introduction, when answering the question 'What is cognition?', let us consider two main groups. First, there are the broad cognitive functions which, it could be argued, are the foundation stones for our function, comprising consciousness, orientation, intellect, psychosocial skills, temperament and personality, energy, drive

Neuropsychology for Occupational Therapists: Cognition in Occupational Performance, Fourth Edition.
Edited by Linda Maskill and Stephanie Tempest.
© 2017 John Wiley & Sons Ltd. Published 2017 by John Wiley & Sons Ltd.
Companion Website: www.wiley.com/go/maskill/neuropsychologyOT

and sleep (WHO 2001). Second, there are specific cognitive modalities, the building blocks for our function, comprising attention, memory, psychomotor functions, emotions, perceptual skills across all the senses, higher level skills (executive functioning), praxis and experience of self and time (WHO 2001). Our ability to interact in a meaningful way, within our environment, is dependent on a complex interplay of these skills.

The Functional and Social Impact of Cognitive Impairments

The impact of cognitive impairments on the individual, their partners, family and friends can be significant. The lived experience allows us some insight into the real story.

The lived experience of cognitive impairments (adapted from Erikson and Tham 2010; Gelech and Desjardins 2011; Lorenz 2010)

I can get tired, irritable and worried because basic activities need more energy, planning and attention. These difficulties have persisted and sometimes I feel out of control. I wonder about the sort of person I have become but I recognise my old self when I do my previous occupations: 'I am a customer; yes I can be that for a while'. I use tricks so I can remember to do things like setting the table; sometimes I need them but not always.

Living with the effects of brain injury is like living in a fog; sometimes my head is scrambled and the shell of my life is broken. I think about my lost dreams and feel the chaos of my daily life. But I compensate for this; I put labels on things, I use a timetable and all the time I'm developing a new identity.

I'm building a new self now, with elements of my old self and new bits, some are good and some are not so good. But I need to accept the death of my old self.

The need for cognitive rehabilitation may be self-evident. But there is debate about what it is and the contributions made by occupational therapy. Within all forms of rehabilitation, models and frameworks help us to conceptualise the processes involved (Wilson 2002) and to think about how and why we should assess, intervene and evaluate. Of great importance is that they help us, as therapists, to understand and articulate the impact of, for example, cognitive impairments on an individual and their family.

To this end, Chapter 1 will start with a brief debate on what comprises cognitive rehabilitation and the unique role for occupational therapy within the process. Specific theoretical frameworks and models will be described in terms of their usefulness to aid our clinical reasoning and then applied to the occupational therapy process, to demonstrate the need to embed our clinical practice within the theory base. Finally, this chapter will summarise why it is essential for occupational therapists to understand the nature of cognitive impairments.

The Scope of Cognitive Rehabilitation

Cognitive rehabilitation draws upon theories from a number of disciplines including neuropsychology, occupational therapy, speech and language therapy and special education; therefore it is not the exclusive domain of one profession. A single definition of cognitive rehabilitation remains elusive; indeed, it has been questioned whether the term itself should be replaced by 'rehabilitation of individuals with cognitive impairments' (Sohlberg and Mateer 2001). This is of particular relevance to occupational therapists where the focus of rehabilitation belongs with the individuals in their context, rather than 'treating' impairments per se.

But Wilson (2002) argues that, in its broadest sense, cognitive rehabilitation should be defined as a process which focuses on real-life, functional problems and is collaborative, involving the individual, their relatives, the multidisciplinary team and the wider community.

In his seminal paper, in 1947, Oliver Zangwill (an influential British neuropsychologist) also spoke about the need to 'join forces' for the rehabilitation of psychological aspects in cases of brain injury. He outlined three activities comprising the scope of psychological rehabilitation: compensation, substitution and direct training. They are worthy of a brief exploration here as the different levels of intervention proposed by Zangwill (1947) resonate with current clinical practice, as will be explored further in Chapter 3. Zangwill defines direct retraining as an attempt to re-educate and remediate the actual impairment, more successful, he noted, in physical aspects of therapy. Substitution seeks to offer an alternative solution to solve the problem but in practice is likely to be a refined version of the final activity. Compensation aims to introduce new internal or external approaches to solve problems, despite the persistence of the underlying impairment.

Current evidence-based guidelines support comprehensive holistic rehabilitation using compensatory strategies, including Zangwill's concept of substitution, to manage the risks associated with cognitive impairments in multiple sclerosis (NICE 2014); to help people with their occupational performance post stroke (Gillen *et al.* 2014); or to compensate for any impairment affecting activities or safety (Intercollegiate Stroke Working Party 2016).

Cognitive Rehabilitation and the Role of Occupational Therapy

Occupation is defined as a 'group of activities that has personal and sociocultural meaning, is named within a culture and supports participation in society. Occupations can be categorised as self-care, productivity and/or leisure' (Creek 2010). But there are a number of definitions to expand upon and challenge our understanding of occupation in the literature, a debate of which is beyond the scope of this text. However, at the heart of the concept is the understanding that occupations are everything people do to occupy themselves while contributing to the communities in which they live (Law *et al.* 1997, p. 32).

That any health problem can have implications for all aspects of life, and not just the physical and mental state of the individual, is now an accepted view. It is endorsed and embodied within the World Health Organisation's definition of health (1946) as: '... a state of complete physical, mental and social well-being and not merely the absence of disease or infirmity.'

By accepting the definitions of occupation and health given above, it can be appreciated that the occupational components of an individual's life become central to health and well-being.

For individuals with neurological damage, cognitive impairments are often the source of functional problems but they are unseen, difficult to manage or misunderstood. Poor task performance, in the absence of motor deficits, may originate in poor object recognition or an inability to sequence. The man who cannot recognise his partner's face may be mistakenly labelled with memory loss rather than prosopagnosia. The older woman who does not respond to questions may have an attention problem which is often confused with deafness. Also there are several possible reasons which may account for a previously independent widower, who lives alone, being unable to organise his daily routine.

Disorders of brain structure or function, inherited or acquired, may give rise to difficulties in the ways in which people think, feel and/or act. These difficulties can cause loss of, or difficulties in, the abilities to acquire or maintain skills. This results in changes in the social, economic and home circumstances of the individual and his family, some of which were outlined in 'The lived experience', above. Within the context of occupation, cognitive deficits are likely to impact on some, if not all, aspects of life. Occupational therapy forms a significant component of rehabilitation.

Occupational therapists engage with people as patients, clients, students, workers and family members, in a range of environments such as hospitals, community resource centres, schools, the workplace and the home. Hence, occupational assessment becomes paramount to investigate the full impact of cognitive deficits upon the life of the affected individual, and also upon the people with whom he/she relates and interacts.

The scope of cognitive rehabilitation arguably embraces virtually all aspects of life. Assessment is only one part of a process that seeks to enable an individual to function optimally within his or her usual environment(s), to maintain health and well-being, and engage in valued occupations (Crepeau *et al.* 2003). The causes (for example, traumatic brain injury, cerebrovascular disease, infection) and the nature of cognitive deficits may require intermittent or long-term engagement with rehabilitation and/or support services, at any point in life.

Cognition, Occupation and the International Classification of Functioning, Disability and Health

Effective therapeutic intervention requires a means of gathering and organising information (a framework). This needs to address not only neurological functioning but also the individual's capacity for and ability to engage and participate in necessary and valued occupations. It requires the means to address the interrelationship of the person and his occupations with the environments and contexts in which they occur.

Occupational therapists have become accustomed to working within frameworks derived from theoretical models of practice and profession-specific theories of human occupation. In parallel, since 2001, the World Health Organisation (WHO) endorsed a framework and detailed classification for the description of all aspects of health and related factors, for use across a range of organisations and within multi-disciplinary teams.

The International Classification of Functioning, Disability and Health (ICF) (WHO 2001) is a multipurpose system of classification developed through international collaboration, including disability rights groups and carer organisations, that codifies health and health-related aspects of human life. Its chief aim is to provide a common language of concepts, definitions and terms for examining health and the individual's ability to function within their sociocultural context. It is designed to do so in a way that transcends other unidisciplinary models or frameworks and provides for:

- clear communication between professionals, different agencies, the public and service users
- comparison of data from disparate sources (different countries, different healthcare disciplines);
- systematic coding for health information systems.

In so doing, the ICF also provides a framework for systematic examination and communication of the relationship between disorders of health, the ability to undertake occupations, and the interaction of the individual with the environment.

The ICF is introduced here as a means to facilitate and enhance the assessment, rehabilitation and support of people with cognitive impairments. It is a biopsychosocial framework, as outlined in Figure 1.1, but also a detailed classification that allows a holistic and comprehensive approach to identifying, measuring and intervening with health-related difficulties for any individual, considering health in relation to activities, participation and contextual factors (environment and personal factors).

The use of the ICF has been endorsed by the World Federation of Occupational Therapists, with strong evidence to demonstrate that it has already been adopted by occupational therapists and multidisciplinary teams worldwide (Jelsma 2009; Pettersson *et al.* 2012). The National Clinical Guidelines for Stroke for England and Wales also recommend the framework and classification as a basis for multidisciplinary team (Intercollegiate Stroke Working Party 2016). And, in the UK, the College of Occupational Therapists has utilised the ICF language in the SNOMED clinical terminology OT subsets. SNOMED CT stands for the Systematized Nomenclature of Medicine Clinical Terms; it is available in more than 50 countries and has been adopted as the standard

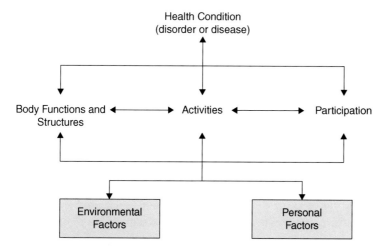

Figure 1.1 The International Classification of Functioning, Disability and Health (ICF). Source: WHO (2001). Reproduced with permission of the World Health Organisation.

clinical terminology for the NHS in England. Further harmonisation between the ICF and SNOMED CT in relation to occupational therapy is planned (Austin 2011). Therefore, the use of the ICF is globally endorsed within our profession, within health and social care teams and between different agencies.

The ICF is structured in two parts. Part 1 classifies and defines body structures and functions, and human activities and participation (in life situations). Part 2 classifies and defines contexts of human function – environmental (external influences) and personal (or internal) influences. The entire classification, which is updated as it evolves, is available to browse online at http://apps.who.int/classifications/icfbrowser/.

Within each component of the ICF, all terms are clearly defined and broken down further. All elements are coded so that, for example, within the component of 'Body functions' we find 'Mental functions: specific mental functions', within which b140 is the code for 'Attention functions' defined as: 'Specific mental functions of focusing on an external stimulus or internal experience for the required period of time'.

Further classification detail is provided for some categories so, returning to the attention example, it is further subdivided into:

b1400 Sustaining attention
b1401 Shifting attention
b1402 Dividing attention
b1403 Sharing attention
b1408 Attention functions, other specified
b1409 Attention functions, unspecified

The ICF in Relation to Occupational Therapy Frameworks

From a rehabilitation perspective, the ICF categorises and codifies all components of a person's life that could be affected by health status, or could in turn have an effect upon health. In the case of people with impairments of cognitive functions, it facilitates the assessment of and intervention planning for consequent activity limitations and participation restrictions. It also enables the exploration of environmental facilitators and barriers within an individual's context. It has been shown to enhance holistic thinking within the stroke multidisciplinary team and clarify team communication and roles (Tempest *et al.* 2013). Therefore, it is an effective framework and classification to use when seeking to raise awareness of the nature and impact of specific cognitive impairments within the multidisciplinary team. But there are limitations, including the as yet unclassified personal factors component, which warrants an occupational therapy-specific model or framework to be used in conjunction.

Within its framework, the ICF includes all those human activities, tasks and roles that conventionally fall within the professional domain of occupational therapists. The UK College of Occupational Therapists (COT) considers the ICF useful to 'shift the concept of health and disability from cause to impact by considering the issues and problems for individuals within their own context rather than by medical diagnosis' (COT 2004, p. 3). In support of this assertion, it can be seen that the classifications used by the ICF usefully parallel current occupational therapy concepts and definitions of humans as occupational beings.

Frameworks of practice utilised by occupational therapists have incorporated large sections of the ICF into their structures, making it possible to translate profession-specific information into, and draw such information out of, this multiagency, multidisciplinary and internationally recognised format. But because of its multipurpose, multiprofessional nature, the ICF cannot and does not seek to incorporate all possible variations upon categorisation of the human state. Therefore, to do this, each healthcare profession will require focus and specificity upon different aspects and will need its own language and concepts.

In short, the ICF is inadequate to articulate everything we do. So, the Occupational Therapy Practice Framework (OTPF), produced by the American Occupational Therapy Association (AOTA 2014), will also be considered.

In contrast to the ICF, the OTPF specifies the need for occupational therapists to analyse activities in terms of their properties and demands upon the individual, as well as the individual's ability to perform the activity. Hence, performance skills, performance patterns and activity demands are components of and demands upon human functioning that do not map neatly onto the ICF framework. However, they reflect the enhanced detail and performance-related information needed by occupational therapists in the analysis of an individual's functional needs and performance difficulties. This further justifies the need to use the ICF, within a multidisciplinary team context, and a profession-specific framework in conjunction with each other. The OTPF articulates the domain/remit of occupational therapy as well as detailing the occupational therapy process as summarised in Figure 1.2.

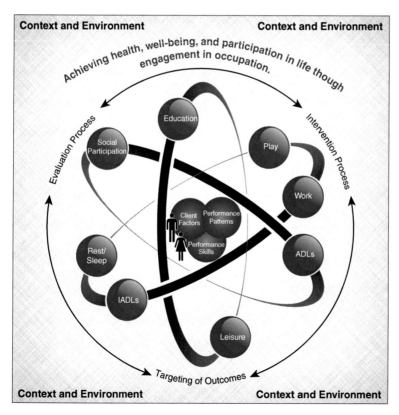

Figure 1.2 Occupational Therapy Practice Framework (OTPF). Source: AOTA (2014). Reproduced with permission of AOTA.

The ICF and the OTPF frameworks will be used to inform our discussions about the role and functions of occupational therapy in cognitive rehabilitation. There are other frameworks that could also be considered, for example, the European Conceptual Framework for Occupational Therapy (Creek 2010). Readers are encouraged to consider which occupational therapy-specific framework or model, in conjunction with the ICF, best meets the needs of their specific clients and services.

Applying Theoretical Frameworks

Most students and practitioners of occupational therapy use a range of theoretical models and frameworks to delineate, organise and understand the occupational needs and problems of the individuals and groups of people with whom they work. The ICF and the OTPF help us to organise large and sometimes disparate amounts of information in a systematic way, and to identify the relationships between them. What these frameworks do not do is provide theories or explanations about why a particular phenomenon or relationship exists, nor do they promote or guide the therapist as to all the tools, methods or techniques they might use to address an individual's occupational needs and problems. These latter functions are served by theories of cognition, rehabilitation and the tenets of the occupational therapy profession. These are explored further in Chapter 3 and throughout Part 2.

The use and value of the ICF and OTPF can be illustrated by a case example. First, the applicability of the ICF will be considered.

Case study

Mr B is a 35-year-old man who sustained a traumatic brain injury when he was knocked off his bicycle by a car. He sustained some soft tissue injuries (bruising and cuts) but these resolved quite quickly. He worked serving customers in a fast food restaurant, and lived with his parents. Mr B was discharged home after two weeks in hospital and referred to the community rehabilitation team which included an occupational therapist. At initial interview, Mr B identified some difficulties with his memory. His parents had observed changes to his behaviour – a lack of initiative in self-care and domestic tasks, and a tendency to be forgetful and easily distracted from the task in hand – which Mr B did not acknowledge. Further specific assessments identified some difficulties with recall and recognition, problem solving, abstract thinking and calculation. Other aspects of cognition, for example short-term memory, sequencing and simple maths skills, were within normal limits.

Activity

Using the ICF framework and classification, organise these cognitive impairments and their implications for occupational performance (activities and participation level) and identify the things in the environment that help (facilitators) or hinder (barriers). See how using the ICF enables us to articulate the relationship between the disability, functioning and the contextual factors of Mr B's life.

Why are Frameworks Useful?

This case study illustrates the use of the ICF framework and classification to identify, systematically, the many interrelated factors, not just the health condition, which impact upon Mr B's occupational performance. From this point the unique skills and knowledge of the occupational therapist are essential to explore, understand and diagnose the interaction of these elements as well as their individual contributions to his difficulties.

In addition to the basic framework of components and definitions, the ICF identifies two components of any individual's activity and participation that together determine his ability; these are termed capacity and performance.

'Capacity' is a qualifier which refers to a person's capability, i.e. their highest or best level of performance in a standardised environment (for example, in a laboratory or rehabilitation kitchen). 'Performance' refers to a person's actual performance within the contexts of his normal environment (for example, in his local shop or his own kitchen). In Mr B's case, he may be able to produce a cooked meal within the familiar environs of his own kitchen, due to being prompted by visual and contextual cues that are present, but may be unable to do so in an unfamiliar rehabilitation kitchen. This highlights the importance of assessing both components of an individual's abilities, as limited capacity for a particular activity would not necessarily predict limited performance. Conversely, successful performance of an activity could not be assumed to indicate normal capacity.

Applying this issue to clinical practice, a neuropsychological test of object recognition might identify a limitation in this cognitive process. This would need further exploration in the person's usual environment and contexts to determine the extent and impact of the deficit on everyday life.

Chapter 2 further considers the debate about assessment at the level of impairment, and whether this is always warranted, if a person does not exhibit any activity limitations or participation restrictions even though impairment may be present.

Why an Occupational Therapy Framework is Important for Effective Rehabilitation

The ICF identifies capacity and performance as dimensions of carrying out activities and participation. It also acknowledges the influence that contexts may have upon the individual's situation (for example, physical environment or economic status) and identifies that these can act as either facilitators or barriers to a person's ability to function (WHO 2001). But beyond the definitions of capacity and performance, the ICF does not offer any further framework for the analysis of human abilities. It does suggest measurement scales for rating levels of impairment, activity limitation and participation restriction, but these are generic and do not allow for describing the nature of a problem in any given area. It allows description of a difficulty but not diagnosis of its precise nature or cause.

Occupational therapists therefore need an occupational framework to further identify and diagnose the precise nature of an individual's occupational difficulties – and strengths – in order to plan effective treatment or other interventions. The OTPF (AOTA 2014) provides a structure by which:

- personal factors, e.g. values, beliefs, body functions of an individual can be further defined

- contextual and environmental aspects can be fully analysed
- performance skills (motor, process and social) and patterns (habits, routines, rituals, roles) a person needs to carry out occupations can be analysed.

Without such knowledge, it would be difficult to analyse fully the impact of any given impairment (of body structure or function) upon an individual's occupational performance. To illustrate this, let us consider the example of driving a car.

Most adults have a general appreciation of what driving a car entails and the skills it requires, whether or not they know how to drive. Most of us, if asked, would identify that driving requires the ability to:

- co-ordinate arms and legs
- see clearly
- know and apply the rules and laws of the road
- operate the controls of a car.

However, what are less obvious are the *demands* the activity makes upon the individual in terms of performance skills, and how contexts can influence these. Such performance skills would include the ability to:

- maintain energy and an effective pace of performance
- sustain attention and selectively attend to important visual, auditory and tactile information
- utilise knowledge (using short-term, procedural and topographical memory) to achieve desired goal (reach destination safely)
- organise self and the immediate environment for effective operation of the car
- initiate, sequence and terminate the tasks involved in driving appropriately
- maintain position and produce co-ordinated sequences of movements, working bilaterally and unilaterally to operate controls
- notice, respond and adjust to changing conditions and unexpected events.

The extent to which these performance skills are needed or used at any time in a period of driving would change according to the context and environment, including the road conditions, local geography and the actions of other road users.

The OTPF identifies performance skills, performance patterns and client factors as being interrelated dimensions, emphasising that it is not only the individual's personal attributes (body structures and functions) that determine ability, but the environment and characteristics of the activity or role itself that are important to its execution. This highlights three things.

- Occupational therapy emphasises performance rather than capacity; that is, the person's ability to 'do' or function in his or her normal environments and contexts.
- Occupational therapists recognise that the nature, content and context of an activity will also influence how it is performed, and therefore affect the demands it makes of an individual.
- When working to resolve a person's occupational difficulties, it is not just the individual's own health and abilities that need to be addressed but also the contextual aspects of his performance, because these may be acting as facilitators or barriers to performance.

Hence, it can be seen that combining the two frameworks provides a systematic mechanism by which the occupational therapist can:

- analyse the characteristics and demands of any given task, activity or occupation
- determine the individual's impairments, activity limitations and participation restrictions that need further investigation and assessment
- determine the individual's residual intact body functions which can be utilised within the therapeutic process to maximise occupational performance
- analyse the impact, both positive and negative, of the individual's physical, social and attitudinal environment.

Why Knowledge of Cognition is Needed for Analysing Occupations, Tasks and Activities

The individual mental functions that constitute cognition involve complex neural mechanisms in themselves (perception or memory, for example), but always operate within a larger complex of integrated and interrelating functions. Perception requires memory because without memory, we would not learn what objects are and therefore not be able to recognise them. Conversely, establishing memories requires perception because without perceptual processing, we could not attach meaning to an experience.

Let us return to the example of driving a car, and think about the activity of driving down a busy street. The driver will need a mental map of the route he is taking. This requires memory and the ability to constantly take in the scene around him and compare it to his 'mental map' (or satellite navigation system), in order to know how far he has got. In other words, he must be able to perceive incoming visual information, integrate it with stored knowledge (or other incoming information) and use this to plan his next actions.

In addition, he must at all times maintain attention to the activity of driving the car – using the controls and checking his speed and position on the road. He must monitor events around him: pedestrians, other vehicles, traffic lights and signs. He may also simultaneously be conversing with a passenger, listening to a radio or disagreeing with his satellite navigation system.

To achieve all this, our driver must be capable of:

- attention – sustained, selective and shifting
- perception – visuospatial, auditory, tactile
- use of working, short-term, procedural and topographical memory
- motor planning and execution of skilled movements (praxis skills)
- executive functions: problem solving and rapid decision making.

This analysis of driving demonstrates the fundamental importance of cognitive processes, their integration and interaction. The earlier example of Mr B also illustrated the importance of individual cognitive functions in daily living, when loss of a single function such as calculation could lead to inability to maintain a job.

Why Knowledge of Impairment is Important

So far, it has been established that knowledge of cognitive processes is important in the analysis of occupational performance and the diagnosis of occupational difficulties (activity limitations and participation restrictions). But it is also important for occupational therapists to go further and be able to differentiate the relative contributions of different cognitive impairments in any given occupational difficulty.

In the case of Mr B, his problems with completing complex tasks could have one or several causative factors.

- Difficulties with recall might prevent him from remembering a set of instructions.
- Problem-solving deficits might result in inability to apply rules to novel problems.
- Lack of drive might mean he is easily discouraged from attempting something that appears difficult.

Knowledge of the possible sources of difficulty enables the therapist to identify which aspects of cognition need assessing, and how to decide upon the best intervention for this dysfunction. If Mr B's difficulty was arising predominantly from his poor recall, then provision of written instructions would enable him to succeed. But if the major difficulty was his problem-solving deficit, it would require intervention that enabled him to learn rules and practise their application in a graded programme of tasks that gradually increased in complexity.

Hence one activity limitation could have several possible causes, and require a different intervention approach depending upon those causes. Selection of intervention without knowledge of cognition, careful occupational analysis and assessment of impairments could result in an unsuccessful outcome.

Putting Knowledge and Frameworks Together

Frameworks such as the ICF and the OTPF provide us with tools to analyse human function, activities and the influence of environment and other contexts upon occupational performance. Skills of activity and occupational analysis provide the means to identify the components of human performance and the demands of the activities in which humans engage. Neuropsychological theories, case studies and research methodology provide an understanding of cognitive systems and their underlying processes. Neuropsychological tests provide health professionals with tools to measure impairments. Occupation-focused tests enable therapists to measure the impact of cognitive impairments on functional performance within specific environments.

When cognitive impairments occur as a result of trauma or disease, the knowledge, skills and tools of neuropsychology may act in combination with frameworks (which help us to structure and organise information) to provide a means to:

- consider the possible nature of cognitive impairments from the location and extent of the brain damage
- screen or specifically test for cognitive impairments
- identify and analyse the cognitive components of activities and occupations
- analyse and assess activity limitations and participation restrictions
- consider and select effective intervention methods and strategies
- determine the outcomes of intervention
- consider the individual's longer term needs within their social context.

SUMMARY

1) Cognitive deficits impact upon every aspect of life and can create difficulties in all areas of occupation. Because of the central role of cognition in human functioning, occupational therapists must have an understanding of cognition, and how cognitive abilities contribute to occupational performance.

2) The World Health Organisation framework and classification of health and health-related states can be used to organise, define and examine the relationships between all areas and levels of human functioning. This includes cognitive functions, their associated body structures and their relationship to human activities and participation. The ICF aids clarity of communication across the neurological multidisciplinary team but on its own is insufficient to articulate what we do as occupational therapists.

3) The concepts incorporated within the ICF make it complementary to and compatible with the OTPF. This is a professional framework that guides occupational therapists in their analysis and understanding of human occupation and occupational performance difficulties.

4) Together with knowledge of cognition and cognitive impairments, these frameworks can be applied, within the clinical reasoning process, to guide comprehensive analysis of occupational performance needs and deficits. This in turn facilitates appropriate and effective assessment of cognitive deficits, intervention planning and outcome measurement.

References

American Occupational Therapy Association (2014) Occupational therapy practice framework: Domain and process, 3rd ed. *American Journal of Occupational Therapy*, **68** (Suppl. 1), S1–S48.

Austin, C. (2011) *Standards for the Structure and Content of Health Records. Supporting Occupational Therapy Practice and Record Keeping*, College of Occupational Therapists, London. Available at: www.cot.co.uk/sites/default/files/general/public/standards-for-the-structure-and-content-of-care-records_0.pdf (accessed 20 September 2016).

College of Occupational Therapists (2004) *Guidance for the Use of the International Classification of Functioning, Disability and Health (ICF) and the Ottawa Charter for Health Promotion in Occupational Therapy Services*, College of Occupational Therapists, London.

Creek, J. (2010) The ENOTHE Terminology Project, in *The Core Concepts of Occupational Therapy*, Jessica Kingsley Publishers, London, pp. 17–31.

Crepeau, E.B., Cohn, E.S. and Schell, B.B. (eds) (2003) *Willard and Spackman's Occupational Therapy*, 10th edn. Lippincott, Williams and Wilkins, Philadelphia.

Erikson, G. and Tham, K. (2010) The meaning of occupational gaps in everyday life in the first year after stroke. *Occupational Therapy Journal of Research: Occupation, Participation and Health*, **30** (4), 184–192.

Gelech, J.M. and Desjardins, M. (2011) I am Many: the reconstruction of self following acquired brain injury. *Qualitative Health Research*, **21** (1), 62–74.

Gillen, G., Nilsen, D.M., Attridge, J. *et al.* (2014) Effectiveness of interventions to improve occupational performance of people with cognitive impairments after stroke: an evidence-based review. *American Journal of Occupational Therapy*, **69**, 1–9.

Intercollegiate Stroke Working Party (2016) *National Clinical Guidelines for Stroke*, 5th edn. Available at: https://www.strokeaudit.org/Guideline/Full-Guideline.aspx (accessed 27th November 2016).

Jelsma, J. (2009) Use of the International Classification of Functioning, Disability and Health: a literature survey. *Journal of Rehabilitation Medicine*, **41**, 1–12.

Law, M., Polatajko, H., Baptiste, W. and Townsend, E. (1997) Core concepts of occupational therapy, in *Enabling Occupation: An Occupational Therapy Perspective* (ed. E. Townsend), Canadian Association of Occupational Therapists, Ottawa, pp. 29–56.

Lorenz, L. (2010) Visual metaphors of living with brain injury: exploring and communicating lived experience with an invisible injury. *Visual Studies*, **25** (3), 210–223.

National Institute for Health and Care Excellence (2014) *Multiple Sclerosis in Adults: Management.* Available at: www.nice.org.uk/guidance/cg186?unlid=2829652272016215203612 (accessed 25 September 2016).

Oxford English Dictionary (2005) Oxford University Press, Oxford.

Pettersson, I., Pettersson, V. and Frisk, M. (2012) ICF from an occupational therapy perspective in adult care: an integrative literature review. *Scandinavian Journal of Occupational Therapy*, **19** (3), 260–273.

Sohlberg, M.M. and Mateer, C.A. (2001) *Cognitive Rehabilitation: An Integrative Neuropsychological Approach*, Guilford Press, New York.

Tempest, S., Harries, P., Kilbride, C. and de Souza, L. (2013) Enhanced clarity and holism: the outcome of implementing the ICF with an acute stroke multidisciplinary team in England. *Disability and Rehabilitation*, **35** (22), 1921–1925.

World Health Organisation (1946) Constitution of the World Health Organisation. Available at: http://ajph.aphapublications.org/doi/pdfplus/10.2105/AJPH.36.11.1315 (accessed 26 September 2016).

World Health Organisation (2001) *International Classification of Functioning, Disability and Health (ICF)*, World Health Organisation, Geneva.

Wilson, B.A. (2002) Towards a comprehensive model of cognitive rehabilitation. *Neuropsychological Rehabilitation*, **12** (2), 97–110.

Zangwill, O.L. (1947) Psychological aspects of rehabilitation in cases of brain injury. *British Journal of Pscyhology*, **37** (2), 60–69.

Assessment and Measuring Change

Linda Maskill and Stephanie Tempest

AIMS
1) To establish the relevance of embedding the assessment process within theory.
2) To describe principles of good practice within the assessment phase of cognitive rehabilitation.
3) To explore and debate levels and types of assessment, including top down, bottom up, standardised and non-standardised.

Introduction to Assessment and Evaluation

The preceding chapter considered the nature of cognitive rehabilitation and the role of theoretical frameworks to guide and structure practice. Two frameworks were introduced as compatible with each other, and aligned with theories and models of occupation, such that their application would promote occupation-focused practice. This chapter will first consider how frameworks link to models and inform assessment and evaluation practices. It will explore the stages and components of assessment, factors that impact upon client performance and types of measurement. The aim is to take a pragmatic approach, still grounded in the theory base, to assessment and evaluation, offering a structure that will guide therapists to appropriate decision making and sound assessment practice.

Linking Conceptual Models and Frameworks to Guide Practice

As discussed in Chapter 1, the Occupational Therapy Practice Framework (OTPF) (AOTA 2014) is a framework of constructs designed to define and guide the activities that constitute occupational therapy in practice. It correlates with the classification and conceptual approach of the International Classification of Functioning, Disability and Health (ICF) (WHO 2001), which is a framework applicable to and overarching all areas of health-related practices. The OTPF also operationalises concepts and theories of several occupational therapy models, for example the Person-Environment-Occupation- Performance (PEOP) model (Baum and Christiansen 2005) and the Canadian Model of Occupational Performance and Engagement

Neuropsychology for Occupational Therapists: Cognition in Occupational Performance, Fourth Edition.
Edited by Linda Maskill and Stephanie Tempest.
© 2017 John Wiley & Sons Ltd. Published 2017 by John Wiley & Sons Ltd.
Companion Website: www.wiley.com/go/maskill/neuropsychologyOT

(CMOP-E) as discussed by Sumsion *et al.* (2011). Both models share characteristics of the client-centred approach and an interactional systems concept of humans as occupational beings. The performance of meaningful occupations is the primary focus of both.

The OTPF can be viewed as a manual for practice, supporting the therapist to be systematic and thorough in defining and analysing occupational performance, and identifying areas of strength and difficulty. Used in conjunction with relevant models, which guide approaches, methods and techniques for assessment, this framework, relating to the ICF, helps therapists to maintain congruence with professional as well as generic principles and values in their work.

Assessment is a fundamental component of any therapeutic interaction between a health professional and client, and is usually the starting point of therapeutic intervention. It involves information gathering, identification of strengths and problems and measurement of the extent of their impact upon the individual within his or her particular life contexts. It paves the way for effective goal planning. Assessment, and reassessment, take place throughout the occupational therapy process, and are used to identify changes in the client's performance over time.

The OTPF organises categories of information geared to the priorities and concerns of the profession, and directs the therapist to consider the relationship of performance skills to tasks, activities and occupations. This guides the therapist as to what information might be elicited through verbal communication (occupational history, needs, etc.), and what is more suitably assessed through observation and measurement (occupational performance and performance skills). The ICF, being a generic framework, provides a comprehensive set of activity domains but it does not differentiate between them in terms of occupational meaning or indicate how they are most effectively assessed.

In this chapter, we will consider the stages and components of the assessment process and explore the factors the occupational therapist must consider in order to conduct thorough, timely and appropriate assessment for intervention planning to meet the occupational and health needs of people with cognitive impairments.

Good Practice in Assessment and Measurement

The following basic principles of good practice should be borne in mind as applying in all assessment and measurement circumstances. These points will be considered in more detail through the chapter.

Considerations of the Client's Fitness to Participate in the Selected Assessment

Do any pre- or co-morbid factors exclude your client from an assessment, for example epilepsy or a history of aggression? Are there any contraindications to its use? Can the client cope with the procedural and performance demands of undergoing this assessment? Are there any communication problems, physical limitations or sensory impairments that will negatively impact on their capacity and performance?

Preparation of the Client and Environment

As with any assessment process, it is important to prepare the client, oneself and the environment (including risk assessment), and at the outset provide appropriate introductions and explanation of the purpose of the session. This is discussed in more detail in the next section.

It is important to determine whether a client fits the criteria for use of a particular assessment – has it been validated for this clinical population/age group/culture? For example, some assessments may assess for cognitive impairments but only for people with stroke, and some may exclude certain age groups.

The therapist must be familiar with the structure and properties of a number of standardised occupation-focused and impairment-level assessments, to assist with the selection of appropriate tools.

Published, well-evaluated assessment tools based upon or related to a generic health framework such as the ICF should always be used wherever possible. This will facilitate effective interprofessional working and communication, and clarity of terms and definitions. The use of uniform concepts and terminology may also reduce the frequency with which professionals need to repeat questions or basic procedures that colleagues have already performed.

Competence in the Use of the Selected Method/Tool

Training may be necessary for the reliable and valid administration of an assessment. If proposing to use only a subsection of an assessment, consider whether this will affect its validity and reliability. If a client shows improvement on an assessment over time, could this be because he is learning how to do the assessment, rather than because his cognitive performance skills are actually improving? Consider the characteristics of the assessment and whether this is a possibility.

Analysing and Using the Results

Be cautious about interpreting results from non-standardised or *ad hoc* assessments (e.g. informal observations, tools developed 'in-house'), as methods are more likely to be of low reliability and unproven validity, and findings may be vulnerable to bias and subjective/judgemental interpretation.

Take care about making predictions from the results of an assessment, unless its predictive power has been evaluated. For example, an impairment-level assessment may not be a reliable indicator of functional performance or able to determine if a person can be discharged home.

Initial Assessment

The most common methods for gathering initial information about a client are by interview and observation. Such initial assessments are exploratory for both the therapist and the client. A checklist of basic information and a protocol of short tasks, to enable preliminary observation of performance, will often be sufficient to make a start on formulating further screening and assessment needs. A standard checklist and protocol grounded in a clear theoretical framework are preferable to something developed *ad hoc* or 'in-house'. Using a published, accepted framework, like the ICF, familiar within and between professions, can facilitate good practice. Interprofessional understanding is enhanced if a framework incorporates all aspects and levels of function, and the concepts are understood by all. Hence, if an area of concern is identified at initial assessment, all members of the team will be able to locate this within the wider health context of the client and understand its relevance.

At initial assessment, it is important to achieve the following.

- Obtain prior information – for example, the client's first language and cultural background, family relationships, educational background and interests, hand dominance, history of the injury/illness and its management to date. Establish the client's current understanding of his health condition.
- Arrange the environment – minimise distractions and ensure comfort, privacy, visibility and safe positioning.
- Exclude confounding factors – drowsy from medication? Infection? Pain? Constipation? Visual impairment – are glasses needed? Is a hearing aid or other communication aid needed?
- Consider the client's ability to cope – can the client sustain attention or meet the demands of the process, will it need to be broken down into a series of shorter sessions, will rest breaks be needed?
- Establish if any sensorimotor, visual or communication impairments are present – assessment results from other health professionals are important sources of information. Often, all members of the multidisciplinary team are concurrently involved in establishing the presence and extent of such impairments so close co-operation and communication are essential.
- Observe any declared precautions or contraindications – instructions such as 'nil by mouth' or manual handling directives could directly impact upon the occupational therapy assessment. Similarly, if a client is catheterised or fitted with other medical or surgical equipment, procedures may have to be modified to take these into account.

Making a Start: Initial Interviews

Interviews serve many purposes: helping to establish the basis of the therapist–client relationship; gaining background information; identifying the most effective methods of communication with the client; starting to determine the client's problems, their goals and expectations, and the therapist's role in realising these.

Occupational therapy models and frameworks contribute to the construction of standardised interview tools. Instruments such as the Occupational Circumstances Assessment-Interview Rating Scale version 4 (OCAIRS) (Forsyth *et al*. 2005) and the Canadian Occupational Performance Measure (COPM) (Law *et al*. 2014) explore in detail a person's occupational history, values and concerns. Such instruments require a certain level of functioning for the client to engage with them, not least receptive and expressive communication skills, attention, concentration, memory, a certain level of fatigue resistance and a realistic appreciation of his own capacity and performance (insight).

While such tools become useful in time, it is not advisable to introduce them before the client's ability to cope with them has been determined. Eventually, a tool such as the COPM would be useful for goal setting and measuring progress with the client. It is both an assessment and an outcome measure that can be administered before, during and at the conclusion of treatment. This enables the client to determine goals jointly with the therapist, and evaluate his own progress through therapy. But the COPM is a measure of satisfaction and perception of performance. It does not measure actual functional ability so this example highlights the need to use clinical reasoning to select a range of assessment tools and to be fully cognisant with what they actually measure. The use of standardised instruments will be considered later in this chapter.

Making a Start: Initial Observations

Observation is the other principal way in which information is gathered to help inform the assessment process. When carried out informally, observations have the potential for subjective interpretation and misleading inferences about what is observed. However, initial observations are informal procedures often undertaken during or alongside initial interviews.

Difficulties with task execution can arise for any number of reasons. Proper preparation of the client and the environment as described above can minimise and help to discount possible confounding factors. For example, if a client is asked to reach for a glass and take a drink of water from it, he may experience difficulty if he normally uses a hearing aid but is without it on this occasion. If the therapist is unaware of this sensory impairment, she may observe a delay in task initiation and query receptive aphasia, visual-perceptual impairment or apraxia. Apparent difficulty with following instructions may have nothing to do with cognitive impairment but everything to do with the absence of everyday aids.

Initial observations should incorporate basic, short-term and familiar tasks. As a general rule, complicated and novel tasks make greater cognitive demands and could be beyond the abilities of a client, so there would be little benefit to either client or therapist in attempting these. Tasks that are useful in initial observation include those that can be naturally integrated into the assessment situation. The demands of the task are more likely to be appropriate to context, and this helps to avoid artificial procedures that may have no occupational meaning to the client or for which the purpose might not be understood.

Selection of suitable tasks to be performed during initial assessment will be guided by the client's level of functioning, the environment and the range of cognitive demands the tasks make. The therapist makes use of occupational theory, activity analysis and knowledge of cognition in this process. Depending upon the environment and context (is assessment taking place on a hospital ward, in a therapy department or in the client's own home?), a range of tasks need to be used which collectively make demands of all the elements of cognition. Visual perception, spatial abilities, attention, memory, purposeful movement and executive functions may all be screened to some degree.

It is not possible to select tasks – or indeed to attempt – to assess each component of cognition in isolation. Even basic tasks have multiple cognitive components. The therapist should use tasks that are simple so that, where possible, each makes demands of one cognitive component more than others. Breaking one task down into component stages can achieve the same effect.

Having a selection of everyday items on a table in front of the client will enable the therapist to make a variety of cognitive demands through task selection. For example, items might include magazines, pen and paper, water jug and glass, and a comb. These could be used to ask the client to:

- point to an object – demanding visual perception (figure ground) and object recognition (see Chapter 6)
- pick up the object and move it to another position – demanding spatial abilities

- use or mimic the use of the object – demanding object recognition and praxis
- use two related objects (e.g. pour water into the glass) – demanding all of the above, plus motor planning and sequencing, judgement and prediction.

Note how this sequence of demands is organised so that the most basic comes first, and each task builds upon the successful completion of the others.

Any difficulties with execution of the tasks should be recorded as observed. It is often tempting for a therapist to make inferences about the observation (Mr X could not reach for the glass because ...), but this should be avoided. This is because (a) there is insufficient information at this stage about the extent and nature of the client's impairments to make such inferences, and (b) informal procedures tend to vary between therapists and environments and so the client's performance may be influenced by factors other than his own impairments.

Accurate recording of observations is underpinned by the skill of activity analysis. The form of an occupation refers to how it is carried out (Hocking 2001). An occupational therapist must have knowledge of the performance demands and performance components of an activity in order to observe its form as carried out by the client, and accurately record those aspects that cause difficulty. This includes not only the client's performance skills but also any aspects of the environment that might be supporting or hindering his performance. For example, in the case of the use of items on a table referred to above, the orientation of, or distance between, the client and the table may affect performance. Bear in mind also that personal factors such as cultural conventions may dictate how an activity is executed, and this could appear as unfamiliar, or even abnormal, to the uninformed therapist.

Initial observation is invaluable to screen in an informal way for activity limitations that may be occurring because of cognitive deficits. As emphasised above, one can only describe performance difficulties from such observations, not infer causation. Therefore initial observation can serve two purposes:

- observing the performance of activities may help to indicate the integrity or impairment of component body functions and structures
- observing performance of basic activities will aid prediction of limitations in other areas of occupation and guide decisions on further assessment.

The Outcome of Initial Assessment

Initial assessment should result in the acquisition of basic occupational information and an outline of performance strengths and difficulties. The assessment should record the nature and extent of any observed disruption to task performance, and also note those elements of the task performed effectively.

Further formal screening and assessment may be necessary to fully explore the client's occupational performance and determine the impact of cognitive impairments more accurately. In some cases, an initial assessment reveals no apparent difficulties with task performance but as the client progresses and engages in more complex activities, and resumes roles, deficits may become apparent and the expected level of occupational performance is not achieved. Occasionally, an impairment may be highly specific and only seen in particular circumstances.

Comprehensive Assessment

Approaches to Assessment: Occupation or Impairment Focused?

Decisions about the assessment of clients centre on the relationship between occupational performance, environmental factors (context) and underlying performance components (performance skills, body structures and body functions). The relevant issues are encompassed in the consideration of whether assessment should be 'top down' or 'bottom up'. These are explored by Hocking (2001) and also discussed by Douglas *et al.* (2007) in their study of cognitive assessment approaches and practices of Canadian occupational therapists working with older people.

'Top-down' assessment assumes that occupational performance is the primary measure of a person's ability to function successfully within his environment. All elements, both external to and within the individual (roles, relationships, health, occupational identity, personal needs and priorities, environment), contribute to occupational performance. Assessment is occupation focused, incorporating consideration of all these elements.

'Bottom-up' assessment is based upon the premise that the underlying performance components are key to successful occupational performance. Assessment and treatment of impairments will lead to the correction of occupational performance deficits and there is a direct relationship between impairment and function. Assessment is impairment focused.

A professional consensus has emerged that 'top-down' or occupationally based assessments are most appropriate to the tenets and goals of occupational therapy. However, there are challenges to this view, as presented by Weinstock-Zlotnick and Hinojosa (2004). They argue that the needs of the client must take precedence in selecting a given approach to both assessment and intervention, and identify examples where one or the other may be inappropriate to the nature of the client's health condition or functional difficulty. Evidence increasingly supports the view that impairments of body structure or function do not always equate directly with a given degree of occupational performance deficit, and impairment-level assessments cannot be relied upon alone to predict functional problems (Hocking 2001). Douglas *et al.* (2007) found that their sample of Canadian occupational therapists selected top-down or bottom-up assessment tools for a variety of reasons. For bottom-up tools, these included availability, ease of administration, sensitivity and specificity for screening purposes. For top-down tools, reasons included the identification of performance deficits and predicting safety or need for services. However, top-down assessments were more often non-standardised in nature, which raised issues of effectiveness, reliability and validity (see below 'Ensuring That Assessment is Robust').

Advantages of an occupational or 'top-down' approach can include that:

- the client's experience of assessment is meaningful and is seen to relate directly to his occupational needs
- the relationship between assessment and interventions is clear
- it has a predictive value that can inform discharge and future planning decisions
- the occupational focus encourages the client's motivation and active participation
- assessment tools are more likely to be useful as outcome measures because of their functional content and consideration of context.

Occupation-focused assessment seeks to understand the nature and extent of a client's difficulties from his own perspective, taking into account occupational history, the person's role and responsibilities within the family and wider society, the activities that are necessary and appropriate in his everyday life, what is meaningful to him and what he wants and needs in order to achieve optimal occupational performance. Occupational assessment incorporates both qualitative and quantitative elements: hearing the client's narrative, values and concerns, and observing and measuring functional abilities during activity.

It may be argued that appropriate interventions cannot be planned unless there is a thorough knowledge of the activities and occupations the client needs and wants to perform, an understanding of the contexts within which this person lives or knowledge of basic cognitive abilities required for the performance of activities. Occupation-focused assessment enables the identification of overall goals and delineates areas of function that are a priority, whether that means independence in self-care, the ability to manage a home, reacquisition of work skills or improving general task skills across multiple areas of activity.

Impairment-level assessments continue to have an important, even essential, role within cognitive rehabilitation. Occupational therapists might not always commence the assessment process from an occupational perspective; it may not be possible, or may not address the immediate health needs and priorities of the client. In practice, therapists use a combination of top-down and bottom-up methods according to the needs of the client and the different types of information required by the therapist. Key advantages of bottom-up or impairment-level assessments include:

- confirmation or clarification of a specific cognitive deficit and its severity
- utility for a client who is in a low arousal state and where occupational performance is severely restricted
- monitoring of change over time in specific deficits (remediation effects, spontaneous recovery or deterioration)
- a client finds meaning in understanding the nature and extent of the underlying impairment.

Decisions to change treatment approaches from remedial to adaptive or compensatory can be supported by evidence from bottom-up assessments. For example, repeating a table-top assessment for visual neglect may show no improvement in this impairment, and a decision may be made to teach the client to scan visually during activities, to compensate for this persisting problem. An assessment of activities of daily living (ADL) may show occupational improvement as a consequence.

The OTPF (AOTA 2014) categorises occupations and illustrates the relationship of components of human function to the performance of activities and occupations (Figure 2.1). It is also possible to locate assessment approaches within this framework.

- Impairment-level assessments address functions at the level of client factors and performance skills.
- Occupation and activity-level assessments consider activity performance within areas of occupation.

The nature and content of any given assessment tool can be used to locate it within this framework, helping to ascertain its value and appropriateness within the assessment process, and its relationship to other assessments. For example, the Rivermead Perceptual

	Occupation	Activity/task	Performance skill	Body structure/function
Levels of performance	Example: Self-care (personal activities of daily living) Carries out the activities that enable care of the self safely, independently and appropriate to time, place, context, culture, age, gender	Example: Showering Obtaining and using supplies; soaping, rinsing, and drying body parts; maintaining bathing position; and transferring to and from the shower	Example: Process skills Searches for, locates and selects appropriate object (e.g. shower gel), uses in correct manner, initiates, carries out and terminates actions appropriately Motor skills Interacts with objects and environment appropriately and accurately, positions self relative to task and produces effective movements in sequence	Example: Visuospatial perception Discriminates and identifies visual stimuli – objects and relationships, distance, depth, etc., e.g. shower gel bottle Attention Directs and maintains attention, shifts and shares attention appropriate to task, e.g. Washes whole body Movement Reaches, grasps and retrieves an object
Levels of assessment	Occupational: Performance of whole activities that collectively enable the occupation – in context	Performance of one task or several linked tasks that collectively form an activity, e.g. accessing the shower cubicle, controlling water flow, reaching for and using shower gel	Performance of a task or subtasks, e.g. squeezing gel out of a container. Orientating body to task and adjusting position when necessary	Demonstration of component functions essential for performance at all other levels – identifying and selecting objects appropriate to task, maintaining focus on task, shifting attention then returning, e.g. table-top construction tasks

Occupation	Continuum of assessment	Impairment
←		→
Coherent, meaningful, contextualised Complex, multifactorial Top down		Abstracted from meaningful activity Unidimensional Bottom up

Figure 2.1 Levels of assessment aligned to component levels of occupational performance (aspects of the domain of occupational therapy). Data source: AOTA (2014).

Assessment Battery (RPAB) (Whiting *et al.* 1985) is a test used for people with stroke that screens for perceptual deficits using a series of table-top tasks. It does not utilise familiar everyday activities, and is conducted in a standardised way intended to be the same for every client. It does not seek to measure performance of daily living activities, nor the client's ability to interact with the environment.

The RPAB is an assessment of impairment. Within an occupational therapy assessment process, this tool would contribute valuable diagnostic information for the presence of perceptual deficits, indicating why a daily activity might create problems for a client. The results could guide the selection of adaptive strategies that might help to overcome these problems. The assessment could not provide a measure of occupational ability, nor predict a client's performance of familiar activities in a familiar setting. Hence it would be effective at the level of client factors (body structures and function) and selected performance skills to screen for deficits that might warrant further investigation, or to track possible spontaneous improvement. It could not reliably predict occupational performance. A few studies have found that the RPAB has some predictive value in relation to function. For example, Donnelly's study (2002) found that the RPAB could predict functional performance at discharge when used in conjunction with the Functional Independence Measure. However, the same study also found that the age of the client had an equivalent predictive power.

Not all assessments fit neatly into specific compartments of the framework. Some standardised screening tools utilise activities to assess for discrete cognitive deficits, and therefore serve a dual purpose of measuring aspects of activity performance as well as identifying underlying impairments. The Structured Observational Test of Function (Laver and Powell 1995) and the Assessment of Motor and Process Skills (AMPS 1998) assess both performance of activities and underlying performance skills. As such, they can offer measures of occupational performance as well as identifying and measuring underlying impairments. These types of assessment may help to reduce the overall number of assessments that a client is subjected to and the time taken in the assessment component of the occupational therapy process. However, the clinical utility of an assessment is also influenced by resource factors such as cost, accessibility and training needs, and these may preclude their use in some circumstances and environments.

A thorough cognitive assessment process will incorporate a range of procedures and tools that address all levels of function: occupational performance, activity and task performance, cognitive performance skills and related client factors, relevant to each client's occupational needs. Throughout the assessment process, it is essential that the therapist utilises clinical reasoning to select the most appropriate tools for a given client and situation.

Ensuring That Assessment is Robust

We have considered the choice between occupationally focused assessments and impairment-focused assessments. This choice essentially reflects questions of validity and professional priorities for both therapist and client, i.e. are you assessing that which needs to be assessed in the most appropriate way, which will provide the most useful information for occupational rehabilitation? A further and equally overarching consideration is whether you should use a standardised or non-standardised tool.

This subject has received attention in the rehabilitation literature over a considerable time period. Clive-Lowe (1996) outlined the importance of standardised assessment practices for occupational therapists, not just to ensure accurate assessment of individual clients but also to contribute to the evidence base for practice, enhance service cost-effectiveness and enable accurate clinical audit. Hobart *et al.* (1996) and Wade (2004) emphasised the importance of standardisation to good clinical practice, and discussed the meaning of properties such as reliability, validity, sensitivity and responsiveness. Salter *et al.* considered selection issues in relation to outcome measures for stroke, relating these to the ICF components of body functions (assessment of impairment) (2005a), activity limitations (2005b) and participation restrictions (2005c). Reports of research into assessment tools and practices regularly include discussion of standardised versus non-standardised tool use (Donnelly 2002; Douglas *et al.* 2007). These papers collectively provide a comprehensive overview of factors important in the selection of measurement tools, applicable to cognitive rehabilitation as well as to neurological rehabilitation generally.

A standardised measure is best if you are:

- seeking a measure of capacity (you want to know the best possible level of ability in a standard environment) or of performance (you want to know how the client will be able to perform in his own environment)
- intending to repeat this assessment to monitor progress, or to use it as an outcome measure
- using results of the assessment to contribute to service evaluation/clinical research
- predicting function in another area of activity (the assessment must have undergone research which shows its results are valid for this purpose).

A non-standardised measure may be suitable if you are:

- seeking to solve a problem specific to this client's context
- measuring performance in context, not seeking to predict function in other areas of activity or evaluate potential for transferability of skills
- unable to match the client to the criteria for a standardised assessment
- unable to find a standardised assessment for your specific purpose.

The focus of and priorities for assessment will be driven by multiple factors, in addition to the client's occupational needs and deficits – for example, the role of the service provider and the therapist's work remit within it (acute rehabilitation, community support, respite care, vocational rehabilitation). Government initiatives, policies and guidelines may provide key directives for service priorities. Staff and other resource availability may determine which aspects of assessment are followed through and which are referred on to other agencies.

Whatever the setting, the therapist must select and use robust assessment tools in an appropriate and timely way, in order to provide information of value to the client, therapist and other members of the multidisciplinary team. Figure 2.2 summarises the assessment process, identifying the points at which various types of assessment could be considered.

Which Assessment When?

The diagram in Figure 2.2 suggests that the decision-making process and the order in which types of assessments are used are linear. The dotted line indicates that this may not always be the case. Occupation- and impairment-level assessments may be carried out in parallel, or a client's deficits may be such that some tools such as occupational profiling and goal setting cannot be used prior to functional assessment. Impairments in higher level executive functions may limit the validity of client-centred tools such as the COPM because these functions are essential for the findings of the tool to be valid and reliable; the client needs to be able to appraise his situation. Deficits in global cognitive functions such as attention or memory will limit the client's participation in most activities, and so some assessments may have to be conducted over several sessions, or a standardised tool may not be viable because a client cannot comply with the behavioural demands it makes.

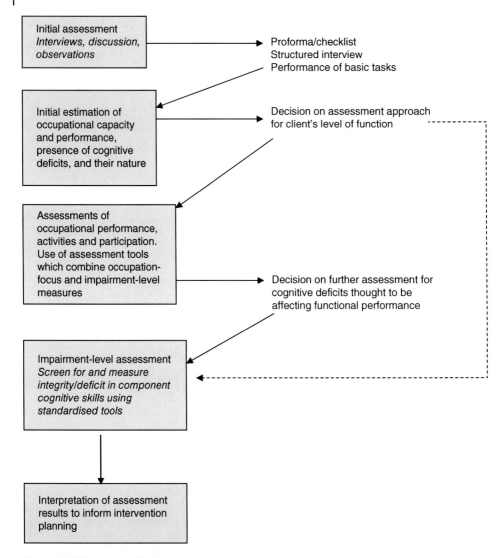

Figure 2.2 The process of selecting assessments.

The perfect assessment tool does not exist, and neither does the perfect assessment protocol. The therapist must use clinical reasoning, underpinned by knowledge and guided by a series of key questions, to arrive at the most suitable choice of assessment methods and tools for each client. All the foregoing considerations addressed in this chapter should be taken into account but finally, the key factors are, arguably, around questions of:

- sensitivity, responsiveness and metric properties of the assessment
- validity of the information collected and reliability of the method used
- availability of suitable assessments:
  - for and with the client
  - for the setting
  - in relation to the therapist's experience and knowledge.

Key Perceptual and Cognitive Assessments Referred to in This Book

A number of key published assessment tools are referred to in this and subsequent chapters, using their abbreviated forms. Below, the assessments are listed with their titles and author (references appear in the reference list at the end of this chapter and may not be given in later chapters). References for other assessments, relevant to specific cognitive impairments, appear in the appropriate chapters.

- AMPS – Assessment of Motor and Process Skills (Fischer 2003).
- COTNAB – Chessington Occupational Therapy Neurological Battery (Tyerman *et al.* 1986)
- LOTCA – Lowenstein Occupational Therapy Cognitive Assessment (Itzkovich *et al.* 2000)
- MMSE – Mini-Mental State Examination (Folstein *et al.* 1975)
- OT-APST – Occupational Therapy Adult Perceptual Screening Test (Cooke *et al.* 2005)
- RPAB – Rivermead Perceptual Assessment Battery (Whiting *et al.* 1985)
- SOTOF – Structured Observational Test of Function (Laver and Powell 1995)
- WAIS – Wechsler Adult Intelligence Scale, 4th edn (Wechsler 2008)

SUMMARY

1) The Occupational Therapy Practice Framework incorporates all components of body function and structures within the ICF, enabling the occupational therapist to use it as a guiding framework in the assessment of cognitive impairments and their impact upon occupational performance.

2) Informal interview and task observations are useful to assist in the initial assessment of a client before more comprehensive and formal assessments are undertaken. Care must be taken in the preparation of the client, selection of suitable tasks and interpretation of findings at this stage.

3) Comprehensive assessment of the client incorporates both occupation-focused and impairment-level approaches, but occupational or 'top-down' assessments could be considered as primary tools. These are most appropriate to the tenets and goals of occupational therapy, but may not always be appropriate to the immediate needs of the client. Impairment-level or 'bottom-up' assessments are essential for investigating underlying cognitive deficits in detail, and to aid decision making in relation to treatment approaches and methods.

4) The assessment process must be robust. This is dependent upon the application of sound clinical reasoning within a clear assessment procedure. Many factors must be taken into account when deciding upon assessment tools; these relate to the client, the service setting, the availability and utility of assessment tools and their properties. This includes such things as reliability, the validity of their findings and the uses to which these findings are put.

References

American Occupational Therapy Association (2014) Occupational therapy practice framework: Domain and process, 3rd ed. *American Journal of Occupational Therapy*, **68** (Suppl. 1), S1–S48.

Assessment of Motor and Process Skills (1998) *AMPS Training Manual*, AMPS UK, Wiltshire.

Baum, M. and Christiansen C.H. (2005) Person-environment-occupation- performance: an occupation-based framework for practice, in *Occupational Therapy: Performance, Participation and Wellbeing* (eds C.H. Christiansen and M. Baum), Slack Inc., New Jersey.

Clive-Lowe, de S. (1996) Outcome measurement, cost-effectiveness and clinical audit: the importance of standardised assessment to occupational therapists in meeting these new demands. *British Journal of Occupational Therapy*, **59** (8), 357–362.

Cooke, D.M., McKenna, K. and Fleming, J. (2005) Development of a standardized occupational therapy screening tool for visual perception in adults. *Scandinavian Journal of Occupational Therapy*, **12** (2), 59–71.

Donnelly, S. (2002) The Rivermead Perceptual Assessment Battery: can it predict functional performance? *Australian Occupational Therapy Journal*, **49**, 71–81.

Douglas, A., Liu, L., Warren, S. and Hopper T. (2007) Cognitive assessments for older adults: which ones are used by Canadian therapists and why? *Canadian Journal of Occupational Therapy*, **74**, 370–381.

Fischer, A. (2003) *Assessment of Motor and Process Skills, Vol 1: Development, Standardisation and Administration Manual*, 5th edn, Three Star Press, Fort Collins, Colorado.

Folstein, M.F., Folstein, S.E. and McHugh, P.R. (1975) 'Mini-mental state'. A practical method for grading the cognitive state of patients for the clinician. *Journal of Psychiatric Research*, **12**, 189–198.

Forsyth, K., Deshpande, S., Kielhofner, G. *et al.* (2005) The Occupational Circumstances Assessment Interview and Rating Scale (OCAIRS) Version 4.0. MOHO Clearinghouse, Chicago.

Hobart, J.C., Lamping, D.L. and Thompson, A.J. (1996) Evaluating neurological outcome measures: the bare essentials. Editorial. *Journal of Neurology, Neurosurgery & Psychiatry*, **60**, 127–130.

Hocking, C. (2001) Implementing occupation-based assessment. *American Journal of Occupational Therapy*, **55** (4), 463–469.

Itzkovich, M., Averbuch, S., Elazar, B. and Katz, N. (2000) *Lowenstein Occupational Therapy Cognitive Assessment (LOTCA) Battery*, 2nd edn, Maddak, Pequannock, New Jersey.

Laver, A.J. and Powell, G. (1995) *The Structured Observational Test of Function*, NFER-Nelson, Windsor.

Law, M., Baptiste, S., Carswell, A., McColl, M.A., Polatajko, H. and Pollock, N. (2014) *Canadian Occupational Performance Measure*, CAOT Publications ACE, Toronto.

Salter, K., Jutai, J.W., Teasell, R., Foley, N.C. and Bitensky, J. (2005a) Issues for selection of outcome measures in stroke rehabilitation: ICF Body Functions. *Disability and Rehabilitation*, **27** (4), 191–207.

Salter, K., Jutai, J.W., Teasell, R., Foley, N.C., Bitensky, J. and Bayley, M. (2005b) Issues for selection of outcome measures in stroke rehabilitation: ICF Activity. *Disability and Rehabilitation*, **27** (6), 315–340.

Salter, K., Jutai, J.W., Teasell, R., Foley, N.C., Bitensky, J. and Bayley, M. (2005c) Issues for selection of outcome measures in stroke rehabilitation: ICF Participation. *Disability and Rehabilitation*, **27** (9), 507–528.

Sumsion, T., Tischler-Draper, L. and Heinicke, S. (2011) Applying the Canadian Model of Occupational Performance, in *Foundations for Practice in Occupational Therapy*, 5th edn (ed. E.A.S. Duncan), Churchill Livingstone/Elsevier, Edinburgh.

Tyerman, R., Tyerman, A., Howard, P. and Hadfield, C. (1986) *Chessington Occupational Therapy Neurological Battery (COTNAB)*, Nottingham Rehabilitation, Nottingham.

Wade, D.T. (2004) Assessment, measurement and data collection tools. Editorial. *Clinical Rehabilitation*, **18**, 233–237.

Wechsler, D. (2008) *Wechsler Adult Intelligence Scale*, 4th edn, NCS Pearson, San Antonio, Texas.

Weinstock-Zlotnick, G. and Hinojosa, J. (2004) Bottom-up or top-down evaluation: is one better than the other? *American Journal of Occupational Therapy*, **58** (5), 594–599.

Whiting, S., Lincoln, N.B., Bhavnani, G. and Cockburn, J. (1985) *The Rivermead Perceptual Assessment Battery*, NFER-Nelson, Windsor.

World Health Organisation (2001) *International Classification of Functioning, Disability and Health*, World Health Organisation, Geneva.

3

Intervention for Cognitive Impairments and Evaluating Outcomes

Linda Maskill and Stephanie Tempest

AIMS

1) To identify factors that will influence the rehabilitation process.
2) To introduce the performance objectives of occupational therapy intervention.
3) To discuss the selection and use of approaches in intervention.
4) To describe methods and techniques used in cognitive rehabilitation.
5) To consider parameters for evaluating the outcomes of intervention.

Occupational therapists draw upon theory, evidence, expert opinion and the tenets of the profession to seek the best possible outcomes for and with their clients. Cerebral injuries often result in cognitive deficits that do not completely resolve, and the therapist must work to minimise the effects of these deficits upon the individual, his occupational performance, and roles within his context and life in general.

Evidence for the effectiveness of particular interventions is growing but remains debatable. As occupational therapists, we must use sound clinical reasoning in the selection and application of interventions, considering the theories and evidence upon which they are based. Just as assessment is an essential stage in planning interventions, so outcome measurement is also crucial to evaluate the impact and effect of interventions and enable professional practice to evolve and develop.

Factors Influencing the Rehabilitation Process

Assumptions Underpinning Practice

A belief in the centrality of occupations to human health and well-being underpins the practice of occupational therapy. It can be argued that the goal of any intervention is to facilitate an ability to live in a home environment as safely and independently as possible,

Neuropsychology for Occupational Therapists: Cognition in Occupational Performance, Fourth Edition.
Edited by Linda Maskill and Stephanie Tempest.
© 2017 John Wiley & Sons Ltd. Published 2017 by John Wiley & Sons Ltd.
Companion Website: www.wiley.com/go/maskill/neuropsychologyOT

to resume former or acquire new life roles and activities, and participate as a valued member of society in whatever way is meaningful to that person in their context. Such a broad-based purpose leads to occupational therapy being a different experience for different people, and its practice varies enormously across service settings. There is a danger that an occupational, or top-down, focus may lead to oversight, or underestimation, of critical performance skills and their constituent body functions that make occupational performance possible. Conversely, excessive focus upon component functions or isolated task performance may result in failure to target interventions to the individual's priorities and unique personal needs. Equally, taking a compensatory approach despite potential for remediation of deficits, or persisting with remediation to the detriment of achieving independence with compensatory interventions, are also risks if therapists are not aware of, or fail to question, the assumptions upon which they base their practice. The preceding chapter considered this in the debate around top-down or bottom-up assessment tools and practices. This chapter revisits the debate in relation to intervention.

As with assessment, intervention should be a judicious balance of attention to the following: body structure and function, performance skills, activity execution and participation needs and the role of the environment (physical, social and attitudinal). A deficit of knowledge and understanding of these mutually interdependent elements, and their relative importance to each individual person, will constrain therapy effectiveness. This may manifest in a 'recipe book' approach to rehabilitation whereby a standard care pathway or standard procedure comes to dictate intervention focus and timings. While valuable in helping to secure consistency and standards of practice, the downside of this is in the potential deskilling of healthcare professionals in terms of reasoning and decision making and, in some cases, a failure to respond to the needs of a given individual. The example of the Liverpool Care Pathway, applied to end-of-life care and subsequently withdrawn in England during 2013–14 due to its inappropriate use, is a case in point (BBC News 2013).

The occupational therapist must utilise interventions that are:

- soundly based upon knowledge of all levels of function, from body structure to occupation and participation, and the context in which a person lives
- derived from analysis and evaluation of published evidence, which may range from expert consensus to findings of randomised controlled trials.

Whether the approach taken is top down, bottom up, restorative, compensatory or a blend of these should be argued on the basis of the client's needs allied to knowledge and evidence, not the therapist's preference or comfort with habitual routines.

Teamworking

The overall goal of rehabilitation is jointly determined with other members of the multidisciplinary team. The team comprises other health and social care professionals and, most importantly, the client himself and relevant others (family members, friends). It may extend to incorporate support staff, residential institutions, voluntary helpers or employers, depending upon the situation and the client's needs. Effective rehabilitation and management require the ability to formulate a clear plan of action and follow it through. Throughout the intervention process, this plan must be reviewed and the client's progress monitored, in consultation with the wider team. Decisions about the focus of intervention, the most effective methods to employ, intensity and frequency of treatment and when to modify interventions will all be influenced to some extent by the opinions of the team and the needs of the client and those close to him. Cognitive rehabilitation can be a long-term process and the team members are likely to change over time as the client's needs change.

Health and Safety

When considering intervention, health and safety is a primary concern. It will determine whether an intervention is feasible, regardless of any potential therapeutic benefit or occupational priority. All health and social care professions encode safety concerns in their ethical and professional codes of conduct (COT 2015). The guidance for preparation for initial assessments given in Chapter 2 applies equally to intervention and treatment sessions, emphasising the safety of the client and of the therapist.

For people with cognitive deficits, the environment can present constant challenges. Disorientation arising from impaired memory or underlying attentional problems may give rise to risk in apparently low-risk situations. Lack of insight into his own health and abilities may lead a client to undertake activities beyond his capacity (for example, trying to get out of bed unaided although unable to bear weight through one leg).

Metacognition: Insight and Self-Awareness

When body structures or functions become damaged and impaired, treatment, recovery and rehabilitation require the active co-operation and participation of the individual. This is one of the central tenets of occupational therapy and rests upon the ability of the person to understand and engage with therapy. This ability stems from many intrapersonal factors, two of which are the degree of insight a person has into their condition and the degree of self-awareness. Unlike damage to other body systems, when the brain sustains damage, these functions may be directly impaired.

Metacognition is the term that encompasses the functions and processes of self-awareness and insight. Both derive from effective executive functioning (see Chapter 10). Metacognitive deficits may result in:

- lack of knowledge of impairments
- difficulty understanding the impact of impairments upon abilities and performance
- inability to effectively direct and adjust thoughts and behaviours to solve problems or to form a realistic appreciation of a situation.

Such deficits will have a major impact upon the effectiveness of rehabilitation and will influence the choice of treatment approaches and methods that might be used.

When a client has full awareness of and insight into his deficits, this can also impact upon his ability to engage with treatment. For example, being unable to remember the way from one place to another (topographical disorientation) or to recognise familiar faces (prosopagnosia) can be distressing, frustrating and embarrassing. Anxiety arising from these experiences may compound a client's difficulties, worsening performance or lowering motivation. It may further impair judgement and lead to poor decision making. Careful preparation, orientation of the client and attention to his safety and comfort will contribute to a sense of emotional security and confidence, and support his ability to engage with interventions.

Time Course and Pattern of Recovery

There are generally recognised time-frames for the different stages and processes of recovery following brain injury. Service provision and therapeutic interventions should match the client's needs and progress as closely as possible. Figure 3.1 illustrates the typical time course and stages in rehabilitation. Variations occur between individuals in the progress made and the services they may access, as well as the eventual outcome of rehabilitation. The nature of therapeutic input must be appropriate to the stage of recovery and progression of the individual.

Determining Performance Objectives of Occupational Therapy

Occupational performance requires the effective use of performance skills, organised into performance patterns, within areas of occupation. These patterns consist of habits, routines, rituals and roles, their individualised nature influenced by personal factors,

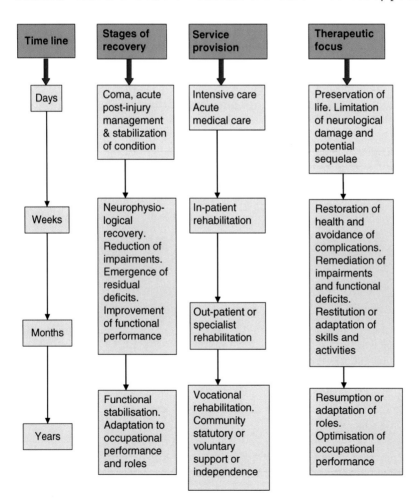

Figure 3.1 Time course of recovery and rehabilitation.

context and environment (AOTA 2014). Knowledge of these influencing factors may be critical to success; for example, the methods and stages of making a cup of tea differ widely across cultures; for some Asian cultures, it is milk based, involves pouring repeatedly from pot to pot to cool it and is always sweetened, which is radically different from the (sadly!) modern English teabag-in-a-mug method. Equally, some routines may have ritual significance and/or religious meaning, hence cultural and religious understanding of clients is important when considering goals, objectives and performance patterns.

An effective programme of intervention incorporates objectives to enable achievement of effective patterns that underpin the ultimate goal of successful and relevant occupational performance. Objectives should incorporate the observable and measurable characteristics of each performance pattern, so that progress towards them can be monitored and evaluated. Monitoring of performance against the objectives for each goal will mark the client's progress and collectively enable review and modification of the intervention programme. Table 3.1 identifies key objectives for cognitive interventions, together with the performance characteristics that indicate their successful achievement. These can be applied to any given task or activity that forms a focus of intervention.

The table illustrates that each aspect of performance (habit – routine – ritual – role) (AOTA 2014) builds upon characteristics of the preceding one, and with each successive aspect, the complexity of demands upon cognition increases. Habitual performance is

Table 3.1 Performance objectives of occupational interventions.

Performance pattern	Performance objective (what is to be achieved)	Characteristics of performance (what indicates that the objective is being achieved?)
Habits	Automatic execution of tasks	Consistent sequence of actions Consistent use of tools Within a consistent environment
Routines	Performance of tasks in an established sequence Able to transfer performance to other similar environments	Logical order Context appropriate Time appropriate Transferable
Rituals	As with routines (above), but performed according to established practice within a social/cultural/religious and usually temporal context, e.g. attending Friday prayers, giving a speech, buying, wrapping and giving Christmas gifts. Overlaps with role characteristics (below)	As with routines, above, but may also include specific requirements of dress, speech and/or objects, rigid adherence to temporal parameters and/or social and physical behaviours. Overlaps with role characteristics (below)
Roles	Performance of activities incorporating a variety of tasks, in variable contexts	Consistent and appropriate execution of tasks and activities in sequence and according to context. Transferable and generalisable to a range of environments Able to adapt in novel situations

characterised by automatic behaviours. Routines require a combination of automaticity with transferability. Rituals carry symbolic, cultural or religious meaning and may be closely tied to role, personal routine or set contexts or periods of time. Role performance requires the ability to apply a range of strategies in varying contexts with a range of demands. Each makes increasing demands upon problem solving and other executive functions. Intervention should address the level of performance at which the client begins to exhibit difficulty. For example, seeking to remediate the performance of routines if habits are not established will impose demands upon the client in excess of abilities. This will result at best in unsuccessful intervention, and at worst in non-co-operation and disengagement of the client.

Selecting and Using Therapeutic Approaches

What is an Approach?

The professional taxonomy of occupational therapy can be confusing. Some terms are used interchangeably in the published literature. For example, the ICF is referred to in this book, and by the World Health Organisation (WHO 2001), as a framework. It is referred to by the College of Occupational Therapists as both a framework and a model (COT 2004), and by some authors (e.g. Bilbao *et al.* 2003) as a model. Within the field of cognitive rehabilitation, the terms 'approach' and 'model' also seem to be used interchangeably (Lee *et al.* 2001).

In brief, models and frameworks form bases upon which to organise and prioritise information about a client and identify treatment needs, as we have seen in Chapter 2. The term 'approach' concerns how a model or framework is put into operation in interventions. An approach usually derives from one or more related theories and specifies how problems (impairments, activity limitations) should be dealt with. Quite often, a therapist will select and use several approaches with a client in order to address a range of problems or to meet needs as they change over time.

Within cognitive rehabilitation, approaches to intervention have traditionally fallen into one of two categories: remedial and adaptive. Occupational therapists utilise both but are concerned with the ability of the client to perform within his own life and environmental contexts, and with the meanings and values the client holds for his activities, occupations and roles. This has led to the formulation of a third, functional, approach.

The Remedial/Restorative Approach

The remedial approach aims to restore and improve impaired functions by supporting and facilitating the brain's capacity for recovery and plasticity. This approach is derived from theories of recovery from cerebral injury. It assumes a capacity for recovery of functions, through such processes as axonal sprouting, synaptic plasticity and reorganisation of function in which undamaged areas of the brain take over functions of damaged areas. Treatment methods aimed at improving specific impairments (e.g. memory training, table-top perceptual exercises) are hypothesised to result in improvement of these components, and this in turn will lead to improvement in functional performance.

The Adaptive/Compensatory Approach

This approach recognises that cognitive impairments frequently persist to some degree following cerebral injury, based upon the premise that recovery within the central nervous system is limited. The focus is upon optimising remaining functions and utilising the person's capacity for learning new strategies and techniques to overcome difficulties. This also incorporates manipulation of the environment to meet the person's needs. Improvement in functional abilities is sought through the use of strategies and techniques to compensate for impairments. Treatment methods utilise theories of learning and may involve adaptation of activities or of the environment to compensate for persisting limitations and optimise independence. In the case of a person with persistent deficits of figure-ground discrimination, the use of bright colours to differentiate crockery would help to locate and identify these items in a cluttered kitchen.

Which Approach, When?

Perhaps in contrast to most other health and social care professionals, occupational therapists also characterise their approach in terms of level of intervention, i.e. along the top-down/bottom-up continuum as previously discussed. This introduces another dimension into the reasoning process; not only must we consider whether we are working for improvement or adaptation to a new norm, but also what the best mechanism for achieving either goal might be – a more holistic occupational method or reductive and based on performance skills. Debate about top-down or bottom-up approaches is perhaps less of an issue in intervention than in assessment. We are, after all, *occupational* therapists, and the discussion of intervention methods and techniques that follows will illustrate that there are elements of both these approaches in many of the interventions we construct.

Essentially, rehabilitation, whether restorative or adaptive, reflects the ways in which we all learn as 'normal' healthy individuals, though with methods selected or manipulated to accommodate the needs of the client. Learning is achieved through experience and practice both in real-life contexts and in simulated situations. Equally, skilled task or activity execution is achieved through practice of the whole, and also through practice of component parts. Examples of all these types of intervention will be discussed below and explored further in succeeding chapters.

It is an ethical duty of all health professionals to seek the best outcome for any client. The major objective of interventions is to enable the client to achieve his optimal level of independent functioning in all areas of life, with the best possible health status. The therapist should choose interventions based upon the needs of the client, the evidence for their use and informed clinical reasoning.

Remediation is most often the primary approach used. This is congruent with the aim of recovery and restitution of impaired body structures and functions, particularly in the early stages of recovery from brain injury or other neurological event, when the body's own processes of recovery and repair are most active.

Adaptation can be used either as part of an overall remediation programme or as the predominant approach if a client has reached a plateau in intrinsic recovery and shows no signs of any further progress. Adapting an activity to reduce its cognitive demands upon an individual may be important in the early stages of rehabilitation. As the client's performance improves, the adaptation may be removed to increase the challenge of the activity and bring the client's performance to within normal parameters. In this way, adaptation is used as a technique to grade intervention, within a remedial approach.

Adaptation as an approach may involve adapting the client's environment in preparation for his return home or teaching the use of equipment to compensate for permanent impairments. For example, in the case of memory impairment, a client may use a written timetable or reminders to support daily routines.

The Reality of Practice: Functional and Client-Centred Approaches

Realistically, a therapist will rarely use one approach to the total exclusion of another. The combination of approaches and techniques employed within a rehabilitation programme will derive from assessment and analysis of the client's strengths and difficulties and the nature of the pathology or damage he has sustained.

For a number of years, a 'functional' model of cognitive rehabilitation has been proposed (Lee *et al.* 2001), which argues that occupational therapy interventions are a balance between remedial and adaptive approaches. It is not possible to identify the degree of plasticity and potential for remediation within any one person's central nervous system. Rather than seeking to categorise a client as either having remedial potential or not at any given point in the rehabilitation process, the functional model supports the client-centred view, that performance is the outcome of interplay between external environmental factors and client-related factors. As such, any activity, performed within a context, will have both remedial and adaptive properties. The balance between remediation and adaptation comes from recognising and using each situation as therapeutically as possible, and accurately measuring the client's performance and progress.

Contextual factors facilitate or hinder performance. Evidence for this comes from research into memory and recall (see Chapter 8). Many occupational therapists see this in assessments of people with dementia; a person who is unable to locate items or sequence tasks in the unfamiliar surroundings of an ADL kitchen can undertake the same tasks without difficulty in his own home surroundings. We take cues constantly from the environment in order to act appropriately and effectively. When cues are altered or absent, additional cognitive demands are placed upon us to solve problems, to locate, identify and learn the use of unfamiliar objects or to apply prior knowledge to a new situation (transfer skills).

Knowledge about the role of context in performance enables the occupational therapist to manipulate activities and environments for remediation or adaptation, and to incorporate more or less focus upon top-down or bottom-up elements. The functional approach recognises that basic cognitive processes are involved in every activity and situation; therefore, whether seeking remediation or adaptation, demands are made upon cognition in order to achieve learning and to carry out what has been learned in one or more situations. Again, regardless of approach, all therapeutic interventions require the client to learn, whether it is a case of relearning prior skills and activities, learning new ways to compensate for lost abilities or learning new skills for the first time.

Methods and Techniques in Cognitive Rehabilitation

A wide range of methods and techniques are utilised in cognitive rehabilitation. This section provides an overview and description of the main types. At the end of Chapters 5–11, suggestions are made for the specific application of methods and techniques.

Learning and Teaching: Facilitators and Barriers to Learning

The ability to learn and acquire skills and competence is affected by both external and internal, or client-related, factors. Thorough assessment enables the therapist to identify these, and establish the starting point for intervention.

Client-related factors include:

- attentional level and distractibility
- behavioural difficulties
- sensory processing and perceptual abilities
- fatigue and pain
- sensory or motor impairments
- literacy level
- language and communication skills
- cultural aspects of interaction with others and the environment
- values and goals.

External factors include:

- physical environment – noise, temperature, light, movement and clutter
- behaviour of the therapist
- presence or absence of significant others
- accessibility to comfort needs – toilet, fluids, food.

It is important to recognise the role played by the family and wider social network of the client in a rehabilitation programme. The consequences of brain injury or disease can be devastating to family members, and have emotional, social and economic consequences for all. People are often highly motivated to do whatever possible to assist their loved one's recovery. The family and others may be the most valuable resource of all to the client; the therapist should always seek to engage their active participation.

If a client is not an inpatient, he is likely to spend most of his time in his home environment or perhaps vocational or educational settings. Significant others can be taught how to support, encourage and reinforce what is learned in intervention, or to continue a programme of activity with the client in his own context. In the case of a client returning home with persistent disabilities and dependence needs, the family will have care responsibilities and need preparation and support. Judgement is required as to the impact such roles might have upon family relationships or the extent to which someone might feel able to manage certain tasks or behaviours, but the therapeutic potential is highly valuable and carries benefits for all.

Manipulating the Environment

The environment can be used to influence behaviour and optimise learning. If a client's aggression appears to be made worse by stimuli such as sudden noises or movements, then the environment should be altered to minimise these or prevent the client from being exposed to them. Similarly, if a client is distractible or has visual perception difficulties, a quiet, uncluttered room with minimal visual distractions will facilitate attention and reduce the visual processing demands of the environment.

Behavioural Methods

Meaning and motivation derive from the client's engagement in goal setting. A client with limited insight and executive dysfunction may be unable to identify or formulate long-term goals, may not see any need for them and may have difficulty identifying progress towards them. Behavioural methods may be utilised in which desired behaviour is shaped by positive reinforcement or the gaining of meaningful rewards, relying less on some aspects of the client's executive functioning.

Behavioural methods may also be necessary for clients who exhibit behavioural sequelae associated with brain injury, such as disruption, aggression or disinhibition. Ignoring undesirable behaviours and praising or rewarding appropriate behaviours are some ways of utilising these methods. It is essential that all members of the rehabilitation team adopt the same methods and do so consistently, to ensure that they are effective.

Shaping

Shaping is a behavioural technique. It is used to encourage performance towards an end goal, when that end goal is not immediately achievable. In the early stages, any behaviour which approximates the desired performance is praised or otherwise rewarded, and so the client is encouraged towards behaving in that way. Once a component or level of behaviour has been achieved consistently, praise is no longer given but is given if the next level of behaviour is achieved. Once the desired performance is fully achieved, praise is gradually reduced and stopped. This technique requires that the goal performance or behaviour is analysed and broken down into sequential stages. If several team members are involved in this intervention, all must know what the stages are, which stage the client has reached and be agreed on the form of praise or reward to be given. Accurate record keeping and good communication are essential.

Executive dysfunction (see Chapter 10) can lead to impulsivity and inappropriate behaviour in social situations, such as the use of sexual innuendo or overaffectionate advances to relative strangers. Prompt and frequent praise for acceptable and appropriate behaviour would provide the individual with positive attention and reward, reinforcing it over time.

Cueing

Cueing is a process of guiding and directing performance. If a person is unable to execute a task or activity from prior ability, or is learning a new skill, then guidance can be given as cues. It is important to use cues that are as simple as necessary for the person's level of function, and in a medium that can be most easily processed. Brain damage often results in difficulty processing large or abstract pieces of information and verbal cues should be suitably concise and simple.

Cues can be visual (demonstration), verbal (spoken or written instructions), tactile (guiding or placing a body part) or environmental (for example, colour coding items or areas). They provide the client with information about what to do next in a sequence of actions and improve quality of performance. Cues can be provided throughout a process or only for parts that the person has difficulty with. This technique is useful to grade activity demands as a person's performance improves. Frequent and simple cues provide maximum guidance and support in the early stages of practice, and can help to avoid failure. They can be increased in complexity and/or decreased in frequency until the whole activity is performed without cues. This technique enables simultaneous treatment of more than one problem; for example, while the person is learning to do a task, the form and content of the cues can be adjusted to make varying demands upon attention, sensory processing and memory. Cues are a useful indicator of progress for a client. The form, frequency and content of cues used in the same activity over time can be recorded to provide a record of performance and serve as a measure of outcome.

Chaining

Chaining is a learning technique which can be applied either as forward chaining or backward chaining. The chosen task is broken down into stages. In forward chaining, the client completes the first stage of the task and the therapist completes the remainder. Once the client has mastered this stage, he goes on to complete both the first and second stage and the therapist completes the remaining stages. Gradually, the client completes successive stages until he is undertaking the complete task. In backward chaining, the reverse applies. The therapist completes all stages of the task except the last one, which the client completes. The therapist then completes all but the last two stages, which the client completes, and so on until he is undertaking the whole task. This latter method is useful because it gives the client the experience of completing a task and hence more satisfaction than the forward chaining method. This technique inherently grades a task in terms of duration, energy demands, complexity and information processing skills, gradually building the demands upon the person. Whole sequences of tasks and activities can be chained, and chaining can incorporate cueing to facilitate the gradual increase in a client's functional performance. Deficits of selective attention and distractibility (Chapter 5) can prevent a person from completing tasks successfully, if at all. Backward chaining of routinely performed activities, such as making hot drinks or getting dressed, is a useful form of grading the activity demands. In the early stages, the goal is achieved with minimal opportunities for distraction, and the demands upon attention can be increased to facilitate improved performance over time.

Errorless Learning

Errorless (or error-free) learning requires that the learner only experiences the correct way to undertake a task. The therapist provides instructions, cues or prompts such that no mistakes are made. This method is useful for people who have severe memory impairments or who are learning a task or activity that is to be used within one setting (not required to be transferable or generalisable), such as shaving every morning in the bathroom. Recall of previous performances will not contain erroneous information which might interfere with subsequent attempts. Demands upon problem solving and judgement are minimal as the environment and context of the task performance remain the same. The effectiveness of this method depends largely upon the repetitiveness of the whole task experience. Hence, transferability of the learning is not expected to occur.

Strategy Training

Strategy training seeks to work with a client to enable him to identify his own occupational difficulties, then solve problems, implement and evaluate task-specific cognitive strategies in order to overcome them. The effectiveness of this method lies in the notion that it transcends individual tasks, by working with a client to enable him to apply a technique and improve his ability with a number of activities he finds difficult. Other behavioural techniques are limited to improving occupational performance with a given task, for example drinking from a mug. This method will be discussed further in Chapter 9. It also has roots in the neurodevelopmental frame of reference, with intervention approaches such as the CO-OP (Cognitive Orientation to Occupational Performance) for children with developmental co-ordination disorder.

Patterns of Practice

Brain damage can result in permanent inability to solve problems, inability to transfer skills to other situations, or to develop them into generalised schemas as discussed. Even if high-level cognitive functions are intact, the acquisition or reacquisition of motor skills and task competence requires practice, and intervention programmes must incorporate practice schedules. The most commonly used types of practice schedule are blocked practice and random practice. These techniques arguably provide the most obvious reflection of the differences between top-down and bottom-up approaches to intervention.

Blocked practice correlates to a bottom-up approach. It involves the repetition of the same sequence of actions again and again. Blocks of practice can be chained so that each element in a sequence is rehearsed repeatedly on its own before the whole is put together. Contextual interference is minimal in this situation, as the demands of the action or task remain the same each time. Using blocked practice to learn to throw and catch a ball, one element would be practised repeatedly, then the other, and only after acquisition of each element would the whole sequence of throwing followed by catching be put together.

Random practice more closely reflects a top-down approach. It also involves repetition of the skill or task sequence but with varying contextual demands, such as learning to catch and throw the ball in one sequence. The same schedules could be applied to putting a kettle on for tea; in blocked practice, each stage (picking up the kettle, filling it with water, placing it down and switching it on) would be rehearsed on its own repeatedly while in random practice, the whole sequence would be performed at each repetition. Random practice increases the variability of demands upon performance, as there is increased contextual interference and the need to relate one stage or element to the next.

In terms of learning, some evidence suggests that random practice leads to better retention and transferability of skills, but blocked practice improves performance during the process of acquisition. This evidence is considered in the discussions of interventions for specific cognitive deficits in subsequent chapters. In terms of functional outcome, random practice might be considered more appropriate to the objectives and goals of occupational therapy, but clients with low-level cognitive function may benefit more from blocked practice as it reduces cognitive demands during rehearsal and may provide immediate experience of success. Varying practice schedules as a client progresses is another way of grading intervention.

Feedback and Knowledge of Results

Feedback and knowledge of results are essential to learning. We use intrinsic feedback, information derived via our senses, in the execution of all tasks and activities. We use the knowledge of results of our actions to evaluate their effectiveness, and feedback from our sensory systems to modify and refine our performance. Extrinsic feedback is that provided by others, again as a means of giving knowledge of results or to monitor performance as it progresses. An important element of feedback and knowledge of results is the emotional aspect. The type of feedback we receive from others and from knowledge of results can provide satisfaction, reward and motivation, or disappointment and lack of interest. Feedback is therefore an important therapeutic and learning tool, and is a prominent feature of behavioural methods.

Feedback can be positive or negative, given immediately, delayed, at intervals during a process or as a summary at completion. It may be used to highlight errors, draw attention to aspects of performance, reinforce correct performance and highlight the relationship between actions and their consequences. How effectively a person learns may be determined by the type and pattern of feedback received, both in relation to the nature of the task and in relation to his own personality and the cognitive deficits experienced. Positive verbal feedback given frequently may maintain attention and motivation but if continued over time, may lead to the person relying upon it rather than his own intrinsic systems. This may hinder learning. Feedback given during practice may distract and hinder performance for someone with attention deficits. Feedback given only in summary at the end of a task may be of limited value in the case of short-term memory problems. Again, this points to feedback as another tool for grading interventions.

As a client progresses, feedback may be faded out to encourage consolidation of learning and reliance upon intrinsic feedback mechanisms and personal judgement. Alternatively, interim feedback may be a tactic to challenge attention and test distractibility.

Grading Interventions

Grading is an important tool in the therapist's repertoire. As we have seen in the preceding section, behavioural, learning and teaching methods have inherent properties which allow grading to occur. The 'how', 'when' and 'what' of grading depend entirely upon the needs and progression of the individual client, and so there is no set formula or prescription. In addition to the specific aspects of intervention discussed above, the broader components of a programme or schedule should also be considered as means to alter demands upon the individual or adjust tasks and activities to their needs and capacities. These components are as follows.

- *Time* – the frequency and duration of sessions and activities can be increased or decreased to accommodate or challenge a person's energy levels, endurance and fatigue resistance.
- *Complexity* – contextual interference, environmental demands and the nature of tasks and activities all impose varying demands upon cognitive abilities, and can be manipulated to lessen or increase performance demands.
- *Therapeutic use of self* – the therapist's skills of communication and social skills mean that alongside specific techniques such as cueing and feedback, verbal and non-verbal behaviour can be used to vary the therapeutic relationship as an intervention programme progresses. This might mean adjusting from a leading role to that of an equal participant in the rehabilitation process or shifting decision taking from therapist to client as judgement and insight improve. Empowerment, personal responsibility, respect and choice are basic human rights. Brain damage results in deficits which frequently compromise these fundamental aspects of human existence, and restoring these are the most important, if rarely specified, goal of rehabilitation.

Evaluating the Outcomes of Interventions

Outcomes or Effectiveness?

Just as it is important to identify the nature and type of a person's difficulties in order to plan interventions (assessment), so it is equally important to know the effects and consequences for the person of those interventions (evaluation of outcome). Outcome is perhaps a misnomer. It implies an endpoint and a conclusion, whereas the individual with brain damage continues to live with the impact of that damage upon his quality of life and that of those around him. Outcome measurement is a part of the intervention process which seeks to establish the effectiveness of the intervention, and not to draw a line under the client's progress. This is an important distinction to make, in order to avoid the implication that discharge from a programme of rehabilitation equates to the end of a client's recovery or the end of potential for change.

This discussion concerns the parameters for evaluating outcomes in terms of effectiveness of interventions, as well as the client's progress.

Evaluation for What Purpose?

Evaluation is primarily viewed as a means to measure the client's progress. It is also a vital component in measuring service effectiveness. Every therapist has a duty to provide evidence of personal effectiveness, to contribute to the evidence base for service provision and utilise therapeutic approaches and methods that work. This derives from the ethical obligation to provide the best service to the client and provide best value to stakeholders in the service. Measurement of outcome specifically contributes to audit of service effectiveness and the development of evidence-based practice.

Evaluating the client's progress requires a comparison of performance against predetermined standards. These standards may derive from a range of sources: baseline measures derived from earlier assessments, normative population data, the client's own chosen goals or the measurable objectives devised as part of the intervention plan.

Methods

Reassessment and Baseline Measures

One of the most reliable ways to identify change in a client's abilities over time is to readminister tests or assessments done previously. Assessments used in the early stages of intervention can be used again. This will provide reliable evidence of change if the instrument is standardised. But care must be exercised as to the purpose and validity of repeating an assessment. Occupational goals and objectives relate to functional performance and while an assessment of impairment may show change in that impairment, this may not equate to improved functional performance, as we discussed in Chapter 2. For this reason, in terms of the client's progress there is less emphasis upon measurement of impairment at the end of intervention and more use of functional outcome measures. Functional measures should be selected to provide information that is relevant to the client's current and future occupational performance needs.

From the service perspective, assessing impairments throughout a programme of intervention may provide useful evidence for the pattern or progression of recovery of underlying cognitive deficits. Such evidence, collected from many clients or even across services, could contribute to clinical decision making about when to apply particular approaches or techniques in the recovery process. Functional outcome measures provide information on the levels of independence and performance achieved during the rehabilitation process. They are often key indicators of service outcome and effectiveness.

Comparison to Normative Data

Another form of outcome measurement involves comparing the client's level and quality of function with population norms. For example, standardised tests of time taken to solve problems or don clothing, or of errors made in a particular task, can indicate where a client is positioned within a distribution curve. Such information is rarely of value to a client unless there is a particular reason to know it, for example exploring suitability for a specific job in which performance times and accuracy have to fall within a certain normative range. Comparing client performance to normative data can be of value to services and individuals in researching the efficacy of specific interventions or the extent to which particular cognitive deficits limit recovery.

Goal Attainment

Degree of progression towards a goal can be measured objectively and subjectively, using standardised instruments or non-standardised methods. Objective measures such as observations and standardised functional assessments provide external evidence to demonstrate goal achievement. Subjective measures include the client's own views and opinions of his progress. Together, these not only identify the degree of goal attainment but can indicate the quality of the goal-setting process. An individual therapist, or a service provider, who finds that goals are persistently not achieved, or whose clients are not satisfied with their progress, might use this as evidence of a need to review the goal-setting process.

Goal Attainment Scaling (GAS) is one approach to evaluating goal progress as it seeks to measure the outcome of a given goal against a numerical scale. It relies on the skills of the occupational therapist in working with the client to define suitable goals so is not a replacement for our clinical reasoning. Rather, it provides a uniform approach to assigning value to the goal review process, for example a score of 2+ means the client scored a lot more than expected.

Objectives

Objectives are statements of achievement. They should be measurable, observable and specific, identifying the required components of successful performance (as exemplified in Table 3.1). Written well and in sufficient detail, they form the framework for achievement of each goal within an intervention programme and are useful indicators of progress. For the client, therapist and the service, they provide evidence of goal achievement or the degree of progress a client is making towards a goal. They can be sound adjuncts to standardised outcome measures in providing evidence of client progression.

Patient-Reported Outcome Measures (PROMs)

In recent years, a greater use of Patient-Reported Outcome Measures (PROMs) has been advocated in order to gain a greater understanding of clients' experiences and views. Standardised tools such as the Stroke Impact Scale and the EuroQol EQ-5D have been recommended for use in the UK for people with stroke. In essence, PROMs are tools that can be completed by an individual about themselves, or by a proxy. In some clinical settings, the routine collection of PROMs is mandatory for the commissioning of future services.

SUMMARY

1) In conjunction with Chapters 1 and 2, this chapter has explored the occupational therapy process, with a specific focus upon intervention.

2) A practical approach is taken to intervention, focusing upon the work done with the client, rather than with relevant others. The first section considered factors that impinge upon the occupational therapy process and are likely to shape intervention beyond the needs and goals of the client and therapist. Professional, team and service factors, recovery potential and the wider environmental context will influence the process. Objectives are important in the intervention process, both as markers for progress and for setting the basic structure for goal achievement. The ability to analyse and grade performance is essential for setting appropriate objectives, and the OTPF provides a useful framework.

3) Approaches to intervention are an important consideration. Remediation and adaptation form the two basic components, incorporating top-down and bottom-up methods, but a functional approach that incorporates a combination of elements and approaches is most suited to the purposes of occupational therapy.

4) Learning is central to cognitive rehabilitation, whether the underlying approach has a stronger emphasis on remediation or adaptation. Many internal and external factors can act as barriers and facilitators to learning, and must be considered in every intervention.

5) The family and significant others may play a pivotal role in meeting the rehabilitation and care needs of a client and are essential members of the team.

6) A range of intervention methods and techniques, derived from behavioural and learning theory, form the common components of intervention. Every person experiences the consequences of brain injury differently, and the particular mix of methods and techniques will reflect each person's needs. Consistency of approach and communication between team members, particularly in the use of behavioural methods, are important.

7) Grading is an inherent part of many techniques but general aspects of intervention, the environment and the therapist's behaviour are also useful tools.

8) Evaluating the outcomes of intervention is essential for all those involved. The key parameters for selecting and using different types of measure relate to the needs of the client, the therapist and the service. The use of functional measures enables evaluation of the client's progress and provides data on service outcomes. It is important to emphasise that discharge from a particular service or intervention programme does not mark the end of rehabilitation for the client, but is part of an ongoing process in which change will continue to occur.

References

American Occupational Therapy Association (2014) Occupational therapy practice framework: Domain and process, 3rd ed. *American Journal of Occupational Therapy*, **68** (Suppl. 1), S1–S48.

BBC News (2013) www.bbc.co.uk/news/health-23283820 (accessed 21 September 2016).

Bilbao, A., Kennedy, C., Chatterji, S., Usun, B., Barquero, J.L. and Barth, J.T. (2003) The ICF: applications of the WHO model of functioning, disability and health to brain injury rehabilitation. *NeuroRehabilitation*, **18** (3), 239–250.

College of Occupational Therapists (2004) *Guidance for the Use of the International Classification of Functioning, Disability and Health (ICF) and the Ottawa Charter for Health Promotion in Occupational Therapy Services*, College of Occupational Therapists, London.

College of Occupational Therapists (2015) *Code of Ethics and Professional Conduct.* Available at: https://www.cot.co.uk/sites/default/files/publications/public/CODE-OF-ETHICS-2015.pdf (accessed 30th November 2016).

Lee, S.S., Powell, N. and Esdaile, S. (2001) A functional model of cognitive rehabilitation in occupational therapy. *Canadian Journal of Occupational Therapy*, **68** (1), 41–50.

World Health Organisation (2001) *International Classification of Functioning, Disability and Health (ICF)*, World Health Organisation, Geneva.

Part II

Cognition

Understanding Function and Working with People with Impairments

4

Cognition: Methods and Processes

Linda Maskill and Stephanie Tempest

AIMS

1) To explore cognition, its relationship to perception and its role in everyday function.
2) To discuss theories of perception – top down, bottom up – and their relevance to learning.
3) To consider models of processing in cognitive neuropsychology.
4) To discuss imaging techniques.
5) To provide an overview of brain structures and functions.

What is Cognition?

The information entering the brain from the environment is constantly changing. We adapt to these changes and respond to them by modifying our actions and behaviour. New information entering the system is organised, classified and stored for future use. Stored knowledge from our past experience is retrieved and integrated with the current input. Plans for future action and behaviour are retrieved and activated at the right time and place. Cognition is all the mental processes in the brain concerned with this acquisition and use of knowledge.

The early stage in the processing of sensory information is perception, sometimes defined as 'making sense of the senses'. Perception organises sensory information from the environment into a meaningful whole. All the senses, vision, sound, touch, taste, smell, pain, equilibrium and proprioception, pick up information from the world around us, and from the body. The brain transforms all this input into our immediate experience of the world and our interactions with it. We are usually unaware of perception, and it is very fast acting. However, perception is not simply based on the input that the brain receives via the senses. Our expectations and our past experience have an active influence on perception. Also, what we perceive may be changed by the context in which we see it.

Let us think about a goal-oriented activity, for example making a phone call. Upper limb muscles are activated to lift and hold the phone, while the trunk muscles stabilise

Neuropsychology for Occupational Therapists: Cognition in Occupational Performance, Fourth Edition.
Edited by Linda Maskill and Stephanie Tempest.
© 2017 John Wiley & Sons Ltd. Published 2017 by John Wiley & Sons Ltd.
Companion Website: www.wiley.com/go/maskill/neuropsychologyOT

the body and the larynx produces the speech sounds. At this level of the description, it is easy to forget the cognitive demands of the activity. We can only make a phone call if we know how to navigate through the phone menu, can find the name and number in the address book, activate the call, and if we can both produce and understand spoken words. The cognitive functions in this activity include perception, memory, motor planning and sustained attention. These all co-operate to achieve the goal. For many people with brain damage, it is impairment of cognitive function which acts as the main obstacle to using the phone, even though the advent of mobile phone technology has reduced the demands of this activity. Additionally, think about the higher cognitive demands that are placed upon us when we upgrade our mobile phone and have to attend to using it in a way we took for granted with our previous familiar device.

Theories of Perception

Perception, together with attention, is a basic stage in cognitive processing. We must attend to the features of the environment in order to perceive or make sense of them. In cognitive psychology, there have been two main approaches to the investigation of perception: bottom up and top down.

Bottom-up theories begin with the detailed analysis of the sensory input, and proceed to the integration of all this information with our stored knowledge of past experience. These are known as 'data-driven' or 'stimulus-driven' theories which consider that perception is driven by the sensory information that is available from the environment.

Early processing of the sensory input from a coffee mug, for example, is largely visual, with added tactile and proprioceptive input when we hold the mug. Auditory input is included when the mug is moved around. In the bottom-up theory, sensory processing proceeds through serial stages to higher levels where it is integrated with stored knowledge from past experience.

If perception depended only on bottom-up processing of all the input from the senses, the capacity of the brain would be exceeded. Also, the input from the retinal image may be too ambiguous to form the basis of our visual perception of the world around us. Bottom-up theories do not completely explain the perception of complex features of the environment such as faces.

In contrast, *top-down theories* of perception begin with the stored knowledge of past experience which is compared with the incoming stimuli to the brain. Detailed analysis of all the sensory input is not required, and this means there is economy of the processing demands on the brain. These are also known as 'concept-driven' theories.

At the beginning of the twentieth century, the Gestalt group of psychologists were the first to suggest that a whole object is perceived before its parts. For example, if we see a circle with a short vertical line in the centre and short horizontal line below it, we say this is a face. At the same time, American psychologists introduced the idea that the brain is a dynamic interconnected system and each brain area can assume control for a given behaviour. It followed that the effects of brain damage depend on the extent of the damaged area rather than its location.

Support for the top-down theory of perception came later in the 1930s from Bartlett, who proposed that new perceptual input is compared with items or schemas stored in memory. An appropriate schema is then selected to match the incoming stimulus. This explains why different people perceive the same input in different ways depending on

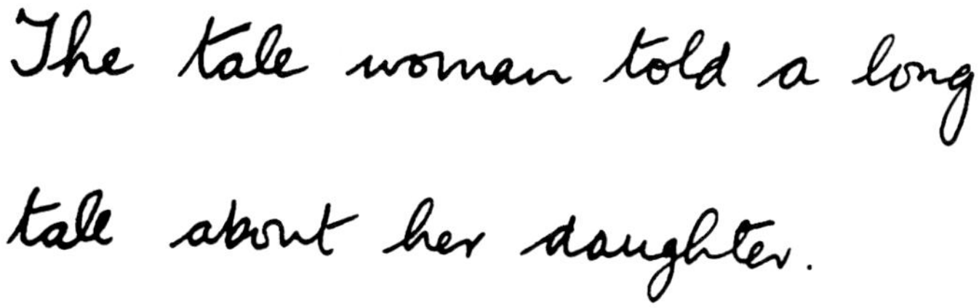

The tale woman told a long

tale about her daughter.

Figure 4.1 Top-down processing.

their experience. Evidence for this is the way we make sense of ambiguous information. In vision, the same input to the retina can be perceived in different ways (Figure 4.1). In this sentence, two of the words present the same pattern to the retina but one is perceived as 'tall' and the other as 'tale'. In sound, the same speech output can be perceived as different. Read aloud the following two sentences:

> That noise makes me want to scream.
> Here is some vanilla ice cream.

The same sensory input can only be perceived in different ways if it is influenced by our stored knowledge, and by the context in which it is presented.

It is generally agreed that perception depends on both bottom-up and top-down processing. We interpret what the senses pick up by integration with past experience. The link between perception and learned experience allows us to adapt behaviour appropriately in response to changes in the sensory input.

In people who have no sensory loss, the functional problems may originate in disordered perception or in the retrieval of stored knowledge related to the task. Normal perception is so spontaneous and automatic that it is difficult to understand the experience of impaired perception in a person with brain damage. While the effects of altered sensory input can be experienced by blindfolding our eyes or plugging our ears, understanding disordered perception is more problematic.

When the sensory input is confusing, we have to make an effort to find a solution. The responses of a group of people to looking at an ambiguous figure illustrate this (Figure 4.2). Some may 'see' it as an old woman, and some may 'see' it as a young woman. After a time, many will 'see' it as either one or the other, or neither and say 'I will believe it when I see it'. It is these exercises that begin to make us realise what it is like for people with perceptual problems; looking at a cup and saucer may require the effort we needed to find a solution to the ambiguous figure.

Cognition in Everyday Function

Cognition is all the mental processes which allow us to perform meaningful activities in everyday living. A large part of our day is spent on activities that are habitual or routine. Some of these support the rhythms of daily life with established procedures while others contribute to satisfaction, for example storing our clothes in an orderly way. Non-routine habits need practice to improve until they become established. Novel situations require planning and problem solving to achieve the desired goal. The cognitive demands of routine and non-routine activities are different.

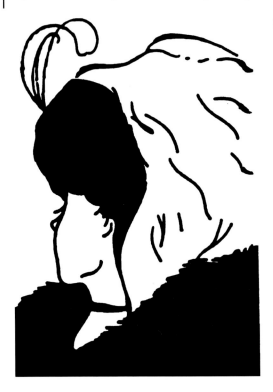

Figure 4.2 Ambiguous figure.

A routine task proceeds automatically with a low level of sustained attention. Most of us have a routine we follow to grab something for breakfast and prepare to leave the house in the morning. If we move house or start a new job, we now have to respond to novel situations in daily living and practice is needed to establish new routines in memory.

Non-routine tasks require an attention control mechanism with focus on a new procedure over time. If we buy a new DVD player or coffee machine, the novel procedure for their use needs extra attention until the routine becomes automatic. Studies of people with brain damage have shown that some may be able to perform routine activities in a familiar environment but are unable to learn new tasks. Others may be unable to organise their day because routine tasks are not triggered by the environment.

Multitasking requires switching of attention from one task to the other. Washing up and listening to a play on the radio are dual tasks that can be performed within the normal limits of attention. When attention capacity is exceeded, errors are made and one or more tasks break down before completion.

Cognition is involved in the planning of actions and behaviours to reach a goal at a future time. If we plan to visit a friend on her birthday, decision making (go by car or bus or walk?) and prospective memory for future actions (go on the right day) are required at the start of the journey. Finding the way involves spatial processing and memory for landmarks on the route we follow. If we choose to go by car and the route is blocked by roadworks, additional cognitive processing is recruited to modify the plan and monitor our progress on the way until we get there.

Stored knowledge about the world is only one part of memory. Skilled actions, depending on the activation of stored procedures for their performance, are developed and improved with time and we become proficient at activities such as touch typing or playing a musical instrument.

Impairment of the cognitive system affects the habits, routines and roles of people with brain damage. Cognitive impairment can have various outcomes in different individuals depending on the focal or global nature of the damage and the person's premorbid lifestyle.

Methods in Neuropsychology

Over the last 70 years, different approaches and techniques have been used to investigate brain function. Each has made a major contribution to our understanding of the brain and the effects of brain damage. This section summarises the methods that have been developed. Examples of the use of each technique will be found in later chapters.

Models of Processing in Cognitive Neuropsychology

One of the milestones in the study of cognition was the development of *cognitive psychology* in the 1960s. This new subject used the methods of experimental psychology to study how normal subjects take in information from the environment, make sense of it and use it (Groome 1999). Experiments are devised to test theories and to develop models of processing in the brain, for example how we store and retrieve information. In these studies, the sensory information entering the brain from the environment under particular conditions is defined and the output response in action and behaviour is recorded. Experiments are devised to isolate the stages of processing between input and output, and test each level. In this way, a model of the stages operating in one component of cognition is developed. Each stage can be considered as groups of neurones firing together, but they may or may not be located in one particular brain area.

In the 1980s, *cognitive neuropsychology* developed as a related discipline which uses the methodology of cognitive psychology to study single persons with brain damage. The methods of cognitive neuropsychology generate flow diagrams of the stages of processing for a component of cognition, for example object recognition or for praxis (see Chapter 9).

Stages and Modules

In the models developed in cognitive neuropsychology, each stage of processing is known as a module, and the flow of information from one module to the next is shown in an information processing diagram. If modules of cognitive processing are independent, it is predicted that each can be selectively impaired. For example, if a person has difficulty in recognising objects, the deficit may be at one of several different levels of processing: basic visual perception, visual structural description, semantic (meaning) representation or lexical (name) representation (Figure 4.3). Tests related to the individual modules in mental processing are devised in cognitive neuropsychology and these are used to identify a deficit in a particular module. For example, tests may show that basic visual perception is intact, but if the person cannot match all the forks in a

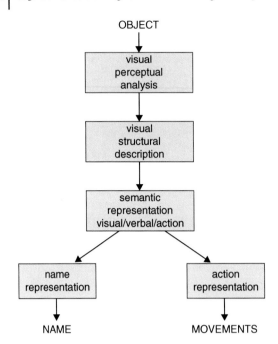

OBJECT

Figure 4.3 Stages in processing, object naming and use.

drawer of mixed cutlery, this suggests impairment in forming the visual structural description of whole objects.

If a person can use objects appropriately but cannot name them, this suggests there are independent modules for the knowledge of the names of familiar objects and for the semantic representation of the function of objects. This is known as *dissociation*. In addition, if a different person can name objects but cannot use them, this is further evidence for separate modules, known as double dissociation.

The following table outlines the stages in the use of objects and the corresponding assessment.

Stage	Assessment
Visual perceptual analysis	Match colours, shapes, sizes
Structural description	Match objects
Semantic representation	Match objects by function
Action output lexicon	Demonstrate the movements for the use of an object

Cognitive neuropsychology has made a large contribution to the understanding of object recognition and language, but some areas of cognition lend themselves less well to the modular approach. When both modular and non-modular components are included in a model of processing, the modules may be co-ordinated by a control unit. An example of this is the model of working memory (see Chapter 8) with separate processing of visuospatial and of speech-based information. The control unit in this model is the central executive which allocates attention between them.

Cognitive neuropsychology is a holistic approach to brain function. There is no particular focus on the brain areas involved and the emphasis is on 'in-depth' study of single cases.

Computer Modelling in Cognitive Science

Cognitive science has implemented computer programs in the study of the cognitive system. A computer program consists of a set of instructions or rules which inform the computer hardware how to perform operations. The stages of information processing in the brain can be separated into a serial flow chart and written as a computer program. The output of the program can then be tested and compared with the response from subjects performing the same operations. In this way, models are developed which simulate cognitive processes in the brain. An example of this approach was used by Marr (1982) in the development of a theory of object recognition. Computer modelling does not mean that the brain works like a computer, but it can establish whether a theoretical process is feasible or not.

Parallel distributed processing, or PDP, and connectionist models are a further development of computer modelling. These models simulate the collaboration of multiple brain regions and emphasise the interconnections between them. Patterns of activity are set up within a network which then 'learns' by using rules to change the interconnections between the nodes of the network. Neural networks learn and store different patterns of processing by repeated presentation of the same input. Connectionist models can be used to predict the effect of brain damage by degrading part of the network and observing the changes in the output of the system. A connectionist network has been compared to a collection of neurones, but the nodes of the network do not have identical properties to synapses, so the analogy can be misleading. Computer modelling supports the holistic approach to cognitive function.

Brain Imaging

The structural and functional organisation of the brain can now be imaged using high-resolution techniques developed over the last 40 years. These techniques are able to reconstruct two- and three-dimensional spatial information about the brain. Imaging has had a major impact on research in neuropsychology.

- *Computed tomography* (CT scan) uses a thin fan-shaped X-ray beam which views a 'slice' of the brain. The X-ray tube revolves round the head of the subject so that the brain is viewed from all angles. The X-rays are absorbed to different degrees by different tissues – less by fluid, more by brain cells and more again by bone. A computer combines all the views and the changes in soft tissue at a lesion site are revealed in a single three-dimensional image (Kolb and Whishaw 2009). CT scans do not indicate functional activity in the brain but they do provide useful information about structural changes. They are used routinely in the diagnosis of neurological disorders.
- *Positron emission tomography* (PET scan) was used extensively over the 1980s to indicate the areas where high levels of brain activity occur by sensing the local rate of blood flow. The subject receives an injection of a solution containing a positron-emitting radioactive isotope which accumulates in the brain in direct proportion to the local blood flow. The results are shown on images of the brain where brighter colours

indicate higher levels of activity. The length of time available for an investigation using PET scanning is limited as the images decay rapidly with time. The subtraction method is used to identify the brain area involved in a particular cognitive function as described in the following example of imitation of movement:

 – *Activation task A* – the subject is asked to imitate specific hand movements made by the experimenter. This produces a scan of the activity of the sensorimotor and cognitive processes of interest.
 – *Baseline task B* – the subject is asked to make predetermined hand movements while watching the experimenter make the same hand movements he performed in task A, but this time the subject does not imitate them.
 – The subtracted scan, A minus B, identifies the brain area specifically associated with imitating movement. PET is useful for studying areas of the brain engaged in normal behaviours (Kolb and Whishaw 2009).

• *Magnetic resonance imaging* (MRI) was originally used to locate soft tissue in the body more clearly than X-rays. In the early 1990s this was developed into functional MRI which, like PET scanning, records the local blood flow in different areas of the brain during activity, but without the invasive introduction of a radioisotope into the body. In this technique, the increase in blood flow in an active brain area is demonstrated by the increase in the level of oxygenated blood flowing through that area. Because it works by detecting electrical charges generated by moving molecules, and the concentrations of such molecules vary according to differences between tissues, MRI enables excellent quality imaging. fMRI has better spatial resolution than PET scans and it can be continued over a longer period of time. With this method, brain activity can be superimposed on anatomy by combining MRI with fMRI (Kolb and Whishaw 2009).

• *Transcranial magnetic stimulation* (TMS) uses a tightly wrapped wire coil encased in an insulated sheath which is positioned over a brain area. A large electrical current is passed through the coil which generates a magnetic field passing through the skin and the skull to stimulate neurones in that area. The effects of TMS are brief and can only be used to explore cortical areas on the surface of the brain.

There are limitations in the use of imaging techniques. A scan may identify an active brain area during a task but the crucial operations may be the specific interactions with other brain areas. Also, the subject has to lie in a scanner, which limits the type of investigation that can be done, and the time course of the investigation is short. These new imaging techniques have extended the knowledge of brain activity related to specific cognitive functions. They are useful to generate hypotheses which can be tested using other methodologies.

Stirling (2002) described neuropsychology as a broad discipline which can be divided into two approaches: clinical psychology, which proceeds from damaged brain to psychological function, and cognitive neuropsychology, which interprets impaired psychological function in terms of models of the stages in information processing in the brain. The methods of brain imaging, computer simulation and investigation of single case studies all contribute to extend our knowledge of the effects of brain damage on function. A clear historical account of the development of neuropsychology, underpinning theories and the approaches and methods of investigation used can be found in Kolb and Whishaw (2009), Chapter 1.

Overview of Brain Structure and Function

With the advent of brain imaging for medical diagnosis and research, knowledge of the neuroanatomy of the brain is becoming more important for communication between the occupational therapist, the neurologist and the clinical psychologist. In this section, the terminology will be outlined, beginning with a brief account of the history of the naming of brain areas and their function.

The phrenologists, in the early nineteenth century, were the first to suggest that the brain was divided into 'organs' or faculties with different intellectual and emotional functions, such as cautiousness, hope, self-esteem, etc. (Figure 4.4). Gall and his many followers believed that a highly developed faculty related to a corresponding large area in the cerebral cortex, and this was revealed as bumps in the skull overlying the relevant area. Later in the same century, postmortem examination of patients with known deficits was used to name areas of the cerebral hemispheres concerned with the production of speech (Broca's area), and receptive aspects of speech and language (Wernicke's area). These discoveries were the first to localise language functions in the left hemisphere.

At the start of the twentieth century, neurologists described clusters of symptoms, known as syndromes, based on detailed observation of the behaviour of people with brain damage. Frontal lobe syndrome was described by Luria who suggested that the frontal lobes monitor and modify action and behaviour. The primary sensory and motor areas of the brain were identified by neurophysiologists in animal experiments and by neurosurgeons exploring the surface of the brain of epileptic patients to find the focus of the seizure.

A detailed system for mapping the areas of the cerebral cortex was developed by Brodmann in 1909. Brodmann identified approximately 52 regions. These numbered areas were defined by the variation in cellular structure and connectivity in different areas of the cerebral cortex. The numbering is not systematic and probably related to the order in which Brodmann explored the cortex. Brodmann's system of numbers is now used in neuroimaging studies of brain function to specify location (Figure 4.5).

Cerebral Hemispheres

Anatomical descriptions divide the brain into fore-, mid- and hindbrain. The largest part, the forebrain or cerebrum, grows out in development to surround the midbrain and part of the hindbrain. The two halves of the cerebrum are the cerebral hemispheres, each with a surface layer of grey matter known as the cerebral cortex. Deep to the cortex, the white matter connects the neurones of the cortex with each other and with other brain areas. The two hemispheres are connected by the corpus callosum, a large body of transverse nerve fibres. This is not the only link between the two hemispheres. People whose corpus callosum was severed to alleviate intractable seizures were able to perform bilateral activities after the surgery.

Each cerebral hemisphere is divided into four lobes named after the bones of the skull which lie over them. Figure 4.6 shows the frontal, parietal, occipital and temporal lobes of the cerebral hemispheres seen in three different views.

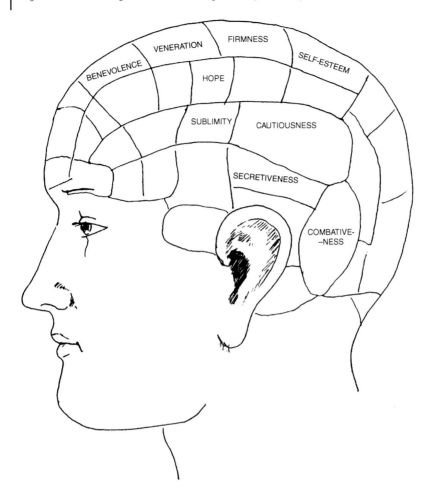

Figure 4.4 Gall's phrenological map.

Frontal Lobe

The frontal lobe, lying in front of the central sulcus, has the major motor areas posteriorly and the prefrontal area anteriorly.

- The motor areas include the primary motor area, receiving input from all the motor and sensory areas of the brain, which produces the motor commands for voluntary movement. The premotor area is important in movements that are externally generated from the changing environment. The supplementary motor area has a role in the initiation of movements that are internally generated. Figure 4.7 shows the position of these motor areas in the frontal lobe.
- The prefrontal area is divided into dorsolateral and ventromedial areas for the purposes of description. On the medial surface of the lobe, the prefrontal area includes the anterior part of the cingulate gyrus (see Figure 4.7b). The prefrontal areas are associated with high-level cognitive processes for the planning, monitoring and

Figure 4.5 Brodmann's cytoarchitectonic map. Source: Ranson (1920).

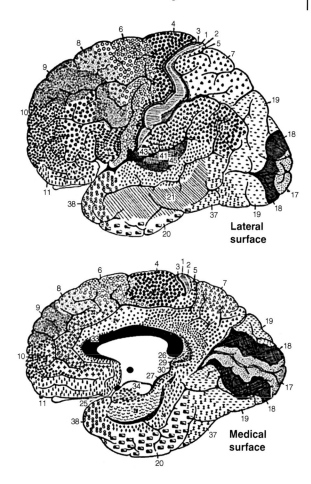

modifying of action and behaviour (see Chapter 10). The prefrontal area also plays an important role in memory.

Parietal Lobe

The parietal lobe lies posterior to the frontal lobe. The somatosensory area, immediately behind the central sulcus, receives touch, pain, temperature and proprioceptive information from all parts of the body. The output from the somatosensory area projects to the posterior parietal cortex for the processing of information about the position of objects in space. A pathway from the visual areas of the occipital lobe projects to the parietal lobe forming the 'where' pathway in object recognition. The parietal lobe is involved in the spatial processing of different areas of space and some aspects of short-term memory.

Occipital Lobe

The primary visual area V1, receiving input originating in the retina of the eyes, lies at the posterior pole of the occipital lobe and extends on to the medial surface around the calcarine sulcus (see Figure 4.7b). This area is also known as the striate cortex due to its

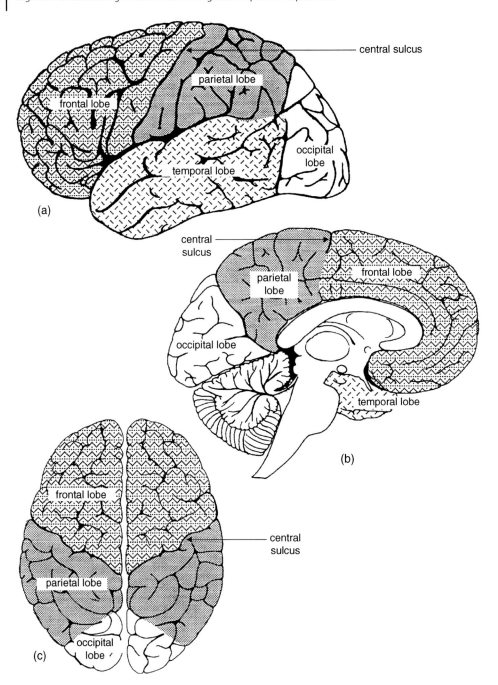

Figure 4.6 The cerebral hemispheres – three views

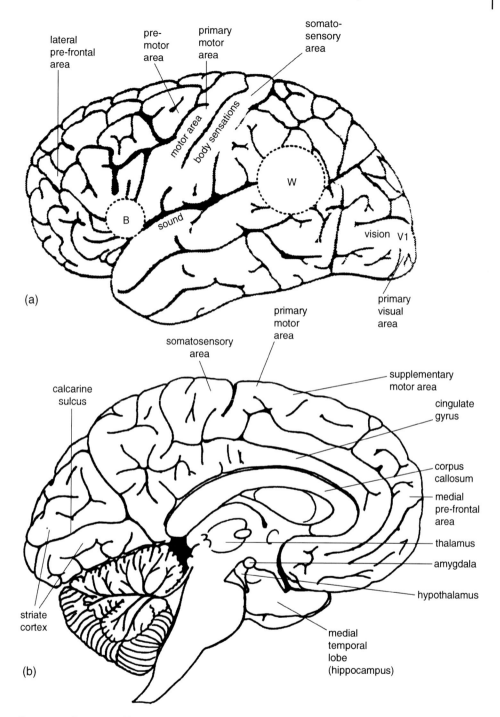

Figure 4.7 Overview of brain areas.

striped appearance. Surrounding the striate cortex is a large extrastriate area which analyses the colour, form, location and motion of visual information.

Temporal Lobe

The auditory cortex A1 lies in the superior part of the temporal lobe, buried within the lateral sulcus with the auditory association area surrounding it. The temporal lobe processes the visual features of objects via projections from V1 in the occipital lobe. This is known as the 'what' pathway in object recognition (see Chapter 6). Each temporal lobe contains a buried gyrus known as the hippocampus because it is shaped like a seahorse. The hippocampus plays an important role in memory and in the orientation of the body for route finding. The area of the parietal-temporal-occipital junction on the left side, known as Wernicke's area, plays a prominent role in language processing, particularly the meaningful content of speech.

Limbic System

The cingulate gyrus, amygdala, anterior thalamus, hypothalamus and hippocampus are all parts of the complex limbic system which can be seen on the medial aspect of the cerebrum and in sagittal sections of the brain. The cingulate gyrus lies on the medial aspect of each cerebral hemisphere, arching over the corpus callosum from anterior to posterior (see Figure 4.7b). This area, together with the prefrontal cortex, plays an important role in the executive functions for the planning and monitoring of action and behaviour. The amygdala processes emotional stimuli independently and also interacts with other brain areas to produce emotional responses.

Right/Left Differences in Processing

The dominant hemisphere, usually the left, tends to be larger and heavier than the non-dominant hemisphere. The inputs to the two sides from the senses and from other brain areas and the spinal cord are largely the same, so any difference between the two must lie in their capacity to process different types of information.

The *left hemisphere*, which is dominant in most people, is central for all language functions: reading, writing, understanding and production of speech. These functions involve the processing of sequences – letter by letter, word by word and so on. The left hemisphere is also associated with the processing of sequences of action, which are the basis of most of our functional movements. For example, in the activity of pouring water from a jug, the actions of reach, grasp, lift, pour, lower and release are performed in series. The sequential processing involved in language, numeracy and movement means that the left hemisphere has been called the 'analyser'.

The non-dominant *right hemisphere* has a greater capacity to process visual and spatial information that cannot be described in words. The recognition of objects, the position of body parts during movement and the spatial relationships of objects and landmarks in the environment are associated with the right hemisphere. The right hemisphere deals with wholes rather than parts and has been called the 'synthesiser'.

Differences in affective processing in the two hemispheres have led to the right hemisphere being called the 'emotional brain'. The right hemisphere processes the emotional information in speech and facial expression. People with right hemisphere damage may show indifference and denial of their disabilities. Those with language problems due to left hemisphere damage often show feelings of anxiety and depression, but they may be able to express and understand emotion in non-linguistic ways, for example facial expression.

The extensive interconnections between all the cortical areas mean that the lobes of the cerebral hemispheres do not function in isolation. Links occur between sensory and motor areas of the cortex; cortical areas to subcortical areas, the brainstem and the spinal cord; and between right and left sides. Furthermore, each component of cognition may involve networks whose elements are located in several different cortical areas. People with disruption in the same brain location can have different outcomes, depending on the extent of cerebral damage and on the other brain areas involved.

Note on Terminology

The terms hemiplegia and hemiparesis are associated with motor and sensory loss as a result of cerebral lesions on one side of the brain. In the organisation of the central nervous system, most of the tracts of nerve fibres between the brain and the spinal cord cross to the opposite side. This means that lesions of the right hemisphere lead to left hemiplegia and left hemisphere lesions lead to right hemiplegia. In the accounts of brain damage in this book, the location of the lesion will be described rather than the side of hemiplegia. It must be emphasised that cognitive deficits resulting from brain damage may occur with or without motor and/or sensory loss.

The Cognitive System

The complex cognitive system functions as a whole, with subsystems interacting at different levels of processing. In order to gain an understanding of cognition, the system can be broken down into components. Each underlying cognitive skill supports effective function and impairment in one subsystem impacts on the system as a whole.

The frameworks for practice classify the client factors that may affect performance in areas of occupation. In the Occupational Therapy Practice Framework (OTPF), the ICF classification for body functions is used, as introduced in Chapter 1. The global and specific mental functions are summarised as follows.

Global mental functions	Specific mental functions
Arousal, orientation	Higher level cognition
Personality	Attention, memory, perception, recognition
Drive, motivation	Concept formation, motor planning
Sleep	Psychomotor responses, emotions
	Body image, self-esteem
	Language, calculation functions

This book will consider arousal and the specific mental functions, drawing on research studies in these areas in neuropsychology. The acquisition of language skills and calculation functions will not be included. Collaboration with speech and language therapists is imperative when there is impairment of language skills and memory.

Research topics in neuropsychology include perception, attention, memory, planning and problem solving. A challenge was issued by Norman (1980) to cognitive psychologists to include culture, consciousness, emotion and belief systems in research into cognition. Since that time, emotion has become a research topic in cognitive science (Gazzaniga *et al.* 2002, Chapter 13) and the way in which attention can operate at both conscious and unconscious levels is an emerging area of research.

The organisation of the chapters in this book is designed to reflect the cognitive abilities that are the concern of occupational therapy practice. The components of cognition will be grouped under the following headings.

- *Visual perception* – object and face recognition
- *Spatial abilities* – constructional skills, body schema, topographical orientation, neglect
- *Attention* – sustained, selective and divided attention
- *Memory* – working memory, long-term memory, everyday memory
- *Purposeful movement* – models of praxis, motor planning, intention
- *Executive functions* – routine and non-routine action and behaviour, the executive system

Chapters 5–10 will address normal cognitive function in each of these areas, together with the related disorders and their effects on function. At the end of each chapter, suggestions for assessment and intervention will be outlined. A final chapter, Chapter 11, will consider the nature and implications for function of mild cognitive impairment. This is being increasingly recognised as present in a range of chronic conditions associated with lifestyle, including diet and physical inactivity, and gives rise to difficulties in daily living. It is of concern because of its relationship to dementia and its prevalence in the older population.

SUMMARY

1) Cognition is all the mental processes concerned with the acquisition and use of knowledge. New information entering the brain is organised and classified. Knowledge is stored and retrieved at a later time. Cognitive processes allow us to interact with each other and with the changing environment, to make decisions and perform meaningful actions and behaviour.

2) In cognitive psychology, theories and models of the stages of the flow of information in the brain have been developed. Cognitive neuropsychology has extended these models based on the study of single cases of people with brain damage. Another approach to the study of cognition uses computer programs which simulate parallel distributed processing.

3) Knowledge of the anatomy of the brain and the associated terminology form a useful basis for the study of cognition and facilitate communication between the members of the multidisciplinary team. The use of CT, PET and fMRI brain imaging techniques for diagnosis and research has allocated function to specific brain areas during the operation of cognitive functions. However, it must be remembered that two people with damage in the same brain area can have different outcomes depending on the size of the lesion and the interaction with other areas.

4) The complex cognitive system can be divided into components for purposes of understanding and to allow the occupational therapist to develop appropriate intervention strategies. Future research will tell us more about the way in which the cognitive components interact.

References

Gazzaniga, M.S., Ivry, R.B. and Mangun, G.R. (2002) *Cognitive Neuroscience. The Biology of the Mind*, W.W. Norton, New York.

Groome, D. (1999) *An Introduction to Cognitive Psychology. Processes and Disorders*, Psychology Press, Hove.

Kolb, B. and Whishaw, I.Q. (2009) *Fundamentals of Human Neuropsychology*, 6th edn. Worth Publishers, New York.

Marr, D. (1982) *Vision: A Computational Investigation into the Human Representation and Processing of Visual Information*. Freeman, San Francisco, California.

Norman, D.A. (1980) Twelve Issues for cognitive science. *Cognitive Science*, **4**, 1–32.

Ranson, S.W. (1920) *Anatomy of the Nervous System*, W.B. Saunders, Philadelphia. Available at: https://en.wikipedia.org/wiki/Korbinian_Brodmann#/media/File:Brodmann-areas.png (accessed 22 September 2016).

Stirling, J. (2002) *Introducing Neuropsychology*, Psychology Press, Hove.

5

Attention

Richard Jefferson and Linda Maskill

AIMS

1) To consider attention within everyday function.
2) To discuss different components of attention: arousal, selective, sustained, shifting, divided.
3) To discuss attentional systems: capacity, networks, goal directed.
4) To consider the nature and impact of impaired attention on function.

The word 'attention' is part of our everyday vocabulary. We 'pay attention to details' or try to 'catch the attention' of a waiter or waitress. This illustrates how familiar we are with attention as part of our actions and behaviour. It is easy to think of attention as seeing and perceiving, but it is much more. Attention, acting early in cognitive processing, both selects the important features in the environment and ignores all the others whilst continuously monitoring the situation for change. The brain selects what to listen to and what to look at from moment to moment. When there are several conversations going on at the same time, we can focus our attention on one of them. However, we may also be monitoring other conversations and react when we hear our own name mentioned.

At times, we are distracted from the focus of our attention by an unexpected stimulus such as a loud bang or a raised voice. Shifting attention to a different location may involve moving the head and eyes or it can be done covertly without eye movement. If the telephone rings, we make a global shift of attention from the task in hand to answering the phone. Shifts of attention are important for flexibility in behaviour and action. Equally, the ability to sustain attention to one thing over a period of time is essential for activity completion.

We perform well-learnt activities on 'autopilot' with low levels of attention processing. If the same activities are performed in a noisy room or in an unfamiliar environment, higher levels of attention are required. Dividing attention between two or more tasks can be done with varying success, depending on the sensory modalities involved

Neuropsychology for Occupational Therapists: Cognition in Occupational Performance, Fourth Edition.
Edited by Linda Maskill and Stephanie Tempest.
© 2017 John Wiley & Sons Ltd. Published 2017 by John Wiley & Sons Ltd.
Companion Website: www.wiley.com/go/maskill/neuropsychologyOT

in each, the familiarity and demand of the actions and the limitations of the brain's attention capacity. Many people can drive while listening to the radio but are unable to do so safely when using their phone, hence the ban on the use of mobiles in some countries. This discrepancy illustrates the differing attentional demands of the two activities. Difficulties often arise when there is a conflict in the same modality, for example auditory challenges when listening to a conversation while following a programme on television.

Attention can be internally generated and reaches consciousness when we focus on thoughts or plans; these can then compete with external stimuli, often resulting in reduced attention. Problem solving and intellectual functions, often referred to as 'executive functioning', all have a large attentional component (see Chapter 10).

Attention processing can be considered as a hierarchy, with each level dependent on a lower one. The basic level is arousal and vigilance, our state of readiness for action. This in turn supports our ability to select relevant information and to shift attention from one focus to another. The highest level is controlled processing, which sustains attention and inhibits competing response choices.

The integrity of the attentional system is considered a prerequisite for the effective functioning of all other cognitive systems, such as memory and executive functions (Penner and Kappos 2006). This suggests it is a cornerstone for cognitive functioning, and is therefore an essential function to assess in the early stages of rehabilitation.

Components of Everyday Attention

Over time, the components of attention have been described in a number of ways, although all of the categorisations reflect its hierarchical nature. For clarity, this section will reflect Sohlberg and Mateer's (2001) classifications and address, in turn, the following attentional components: arousal, selective attention, sustained attention/vigilance, alternating/shifting attention, and divided attention and multitasking. The ICF (WHO 2001) also categorises 'sharing attention', for example when a child and parent are both focused on and attending to the same toy.

Arousal

Arousal is a state of responsiveness to sensory stimulation or excitability resulting from physiological activity in a number of networks, including the prefrontal areas, the ascending reticular activating system and their neurotransmitter systems (Whyte 1992). Tonic arousal is the change in arousal level from sleep to waking, coinciding with the diurnal rhythm. Environmental changes, for example sunlight appearing in the bedroom, stimulate cortical activity and raise the level of arousal to the waking state. The reverse occurs when the stimuli in the environment decrease and we go to sleep.

Phasic arousal is a faster change in arousal, occurring in response to activity demands. The level of arousal depends on the complexity of the task and the environmental conditions. Higher levels of arousal are needed for tasks which use fine motor control or have important decision-making components. Arousal is raised if the environmental stimuli are threatening or a quick response is demanded, for example crossing a busy road.

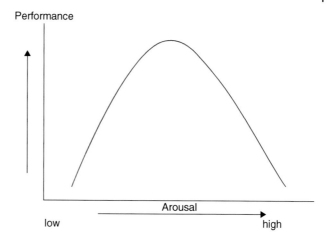

Figure 5.1 Relationship between arousal and performance.

The relationship between arousal and performance is described as an inverted U-shaped curve (Figure 5.1). At extremely low levels of arousal, minimal cortical activity leads to poor response to environmental change and poor motor control. At moderate levels of arousal, we are alert and ready for action. Raising arousal to very high levels leads to disorganised behaviour and, over sustained periods, stress.

Selective Attention

Selective attention is involved in the processing and filtering of relevant information in the presence of irrelevant stimuli (Ries and Marks 2005). The brain is bombarded with information from all over the body and from the environment. If all of it were processed, there would soon be overload of the brain's capacity. Selective attention allows us to deal with what is important and ignore the rest. This leads to the question, 'How do we select the salient features and what happens to all the other input?'. Laboratory experiments in the 1950s, exploring this question, investigated the 'cocktail party phenomenon'. Subjects were presented with two different streams of speech, one to each ear, via headphones. The subjects were asked to attend to one channel only and to repeat what they heard. When there were physical differences between the voices, for example the gender of the speaker or the voice intensity, the subjects were able to attend to the chosen auditory message and repeat aloud what they heard. When the two streams were in the same voice, it was difficult to separate the meaning of the two messages. These early experiments proposed that selection occurs after temporary storage and before any processing for meaning.

Later experiments demonstrated some recall from the unattended channel, suggesting that these are not filtered but are attenuated, like turning down the volume on a radio or TV. The main message gets through with other information attenuated.

The level of processing of the unattended information may depend on whether it is relevant or not and on the perceptual load at the time. When the perceptual load is low, more spare attention capacity is available. Returning to the party analogy, this means our attention can be focused on the other conversations in the room when the present one becomes boring.

Activity

Put on the radio at home and read a textbook or write up lecture/case notes. Make a note of any item on the radio that catches your attention and distracts you from your work. Is it an unusual sound, a known voice on the radio or a favourite tune? How does your experience fit into the theories of selective auditory attention?

(a)   (b)

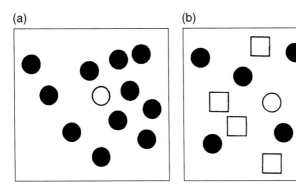

Figure 5.2 Visual search for a target (*white circle*). (a) Single feature – fast and parallel. (b) Conjunction of features – slow and serial.

Next, we will think about selective attention in the visual world, a mechanism by which *looking* is turned into *seeing* (Carrasco 2011). An example of this is scanning the supermarket shelf for a particular packet of cereal; we ignore those we don't like and can selectively attend to and interpret the packaging of the one we want to buy. Various commentators have asserted that attention is selective due to the severe limits on our capacity to process visual information, leading to the concept that stimuli compete for limited resources (Broadbent 1958; Kinchla 1992). Evidence in humans for neural competition has been found using fMRI in which multiple visual stimuli are presented either sequentially or simultaneously. Several studies show that simultaneous presentations evoke weaker responses than sequential presentations, suggesting the presence of competition (Beck and Kastner 2007; Kastner *et al.* 1998).

Early research exploring selective visual attention was undertaken using visual search tasks. In one, subjects were asked to search for a target stimulus in an array of up to 30 distractors and the time to respond to the target was recorded. The visual features of the target, for example shape or colour and the number of distractors, were varied in different trials. When the target and the distractors differed by a single dimension, the response time to the target was fast and it was not affected by the number of distractor stimuli, suggesting a fast parallel selection process. In a second condition, the target was defined by a conjunction of features, for example colour and shape, and one of these features was shared by a variety of distractors. In this circumstance, the response time to the target stimulus was longer and related to the number of distractors in the array. This suggested that attention processing directed a serial search of items, one at a time, until the target was detected (Figure 5.2).

This visual search paradigm can be compared with searching for a friend in a crowd at a railway station. A fast parallel search occurs if he or she is the only person wearing a green jacket amongst a large number of commuters in grey suits. If the crowd is more heterogeneous, additional features such as hairstyle, height and weight are used in a serial search to find the friend and this takes longer if it is a large crowd.

Visual attention provides the 'glue' which allows us to perceive an object rather than a meaningless set of features. There are two forms of processing in which we need visual attention to help us recognise objects: fast parallel processing of single features, for example the colour of the cereal box on the shelf, or slower serial processing of whole objects, for example looking for the whole box (Treisman and Gelade 1980). More recently, developments of the theory have suggested that selection can operate at different levels and visual search is not solely parallel or serial. Studies have shown that searching can be made more efficient by ignoring stimuli that do not share the features of the target. This reflects the real world where distractors are very diverse. There is support for the view that the most important factor in visual search tasks is the degree to which the target can be discriminated from distractors. Focused attention is needed when it is difficult to discriminate between target and non-target stimuli. When the target is easy to discriminate, for example a red sports car in a multistorey car park, a serial car-by-car search is not required to find it.

Further studies of visual and auditory selective attention have considered the role of top-down processing. Desimone and Duncan (1995) suggested that top-down processing in selective attention makes us ready to receive information that is behaviourally relevant at the expense of other input. This has been supported by a number of fMRI studies showing that spatial attention affects the primary visual cortex, which had previously been considered a purely sensory area (Kastner and Ungerleider 2000). This suggests a direct link between the cognitive and sensory systems at an intrinsic level.

There are competing theories regarding how attention is determined:

- past experience directs the detection of priority stimuli while distracting information is inhibited. An example of this is a parent who sleeps through the sound of noisy traffic in the night but always responds to the cries of their baby
- genetically determined.

This latter notion that our attentional systems are hardwired is linked to the importance of survival so that we attend to information that represents a change in the environment. However, this is insufficient as an explanation because we also acquire learned attentional biases through experience – for example on mastering how to read, the letters form meaningful words rather than being attended to purely as shapes.

In summary, selective attention enables us to optimise the performance of a system with limited capacity whilst allowing influence from higher levels to discriminate between the relevance of competing stimuli. Clinically, because selective attention is essential for encoding information into memory, retaining and manipulating information in working memory and successfully executing goal-directed behaviour, a deficit in selective attention could contribute to, or be misinterpreted as, one of the numerous cognitive deficits observed in those living with neurological impairments.

Sustained Attention (Vigilance)

Sustained attention or vigilance is the ability to maintain attention to a single stimulus or task over time (Sohlberg and Mateer 2001) and is intrinsically linked to arousal.

The maximum length of time that an individual can sustain attention is often called the attention span. The level of sustained attention varies widely, even for the same task. In motorway driving, sustained attention over long periods enables us to monitor the road and detect any change that requires action. A warning of a lane closure or the presence of a slow vehicle ahead raises attention to the level required for decision making and response selection.

Alternating or Shifting Attention

Alternating or shifting attention is the ability to switch attention between two or more stimuli or tasks (Sohlberg and Mateer 2001). The focus of our attention is constantly changing in line with the features of the environment and the task in hand. We direct our attention to different locations – to stimuli across the room or the street, to objects and people and to our own bodies. This type of attention is related to the ability to change focus between tasks in a flexible or adaptive manner (Amos 2002), with differing cognitive demands (Sohlberg and Mateer 2001) and is often associated with cognitive flexibility.

Shifting attention occurs in response to a peripheral stimulus, which may be a noise or the sight of a moving figure on the periphery of our visual field. The unexpected sound invokes a reflex movement of the head towards the source of the noise. In vision, attention is grabbed by the moving figure and the eyes move in that direction to bring the image to a focus on the fovea of the retina. These rapid shifts of attention to a new location are automatic and they can happen with or without eye movements. Once attention has been shifted to the new location, top-down processing maintains the focus of attention there. Object-based shifts of attention occur in task performance with multiple objects. Even the simple movement of pouring water from a kettle into a cup involves engaging attention to the kettle and then shifting attention to the cup. In some situations, covert attention shifting occurs, for example while at the cinema we can make way for a person who is late arriving without moving our eyes from the screen. Investigations of attention shifting have described three stages: disengagement, shifting and engaging, each involving different brain areas. Apparent loss of attention shifting in people with brain damage may present as random eye movements, a fixed gaze and an inability to make voluntary eye movements, or contribute towards cognitive inflexibility, depending on the extent and location of the damage.

Activity

This is an observation exercise of passengers on a bus or train. Choose four of the passengers travelling with you on the way to college or work. Take a brief look at people and note the name and location of their focus of attention at that moment, for example a newspaper held in front of them. Next, record any changes in the focus of attention for each person as the journey proceeds.

What was the stimulus for each shift of attention? What was the response?

Note any examples of dividing attention, for example changing track on a smartphone whilst reading a book or looking at the travel information while talking to a friend.

Could you observe any differences in the level of arousal in individuals in this group? Compare your notes with colleagues to build up a profile of the role of attention in this example of everyday living.

Divided Attention and Multitasking

Divided attention is the ability to attend to two or more stimuli or tasks at the same time (Sohlberg and Mateer 2001), often referred to as 'multitasking'. In everyday living, we are often doing more than one thing at a time. Multitasking is a feature of life at work and at home for many people. In this case, we have to divide our attention between two or more competing activities.

Tasks that are regulated by brain networks in closer anatomical proximity will interfere more with each other than tasks controlled by spatially distant regions; this is known as the functional distance hypothesis (Kinsbourne and Hicks 1978). Once again, this suggests that attention is not limitless and therefore at times in competition. Those who subscribe to capacity theories suggest that the brain has multiple processors that can be assigned to different types of incoming stimuli. If two tasks depend on the same resources, the performance decreases for either or both in the event of interference (Leclercq 2002). However, if different processing resources are used for each task, they do not interfere with each other and dual task performance can be as good as when either task is completed alone (Allport *et al.* 1972).

More recent studies on driving performance appear to support these findings, suggesting that driving performance is dependent on the nature of the dual tasks, including the degree to which they share the same sensory modality, and the level of attentional demand. For example, passenger conversation does not adversely affect driving (Drews *et al.* 2008). However, mobile phone use and texting has a progressively more detrimental influence on performance (Drews *et al.* 2009), with drivers conversing on a mobile phone showing signs of inattention blindness, and processing up to 50% less of the information in their environment than a driver who is not engaged in a mobile phone conversation (Strayer *et al.* 2003).

Contemporary orthodoxy has it that the ability to multitask is an admirable skill, leading to improved efficiency. Further exploration of the evidence leads to a more nuanced attitude towards multitasking, recognising that its value is dependent upon the context and activities for which it may be used. The writer Phil Cooke, in a critique of multitasking, suggested that 'the most valuable commodity of the 21st century will be undivided attention'. Some popular assumptions claim that certain people are more or less proficient than others at multitasking, raising the question as to whether there are variations across individuals. These variations may be explained by the influence of practice because, as a task is repeated, the performance improves with practice for both simple and complex tasks such as reading while writing from dictation (Spelke *et al.* 1976). Reporting on more complex work-specific tasks, Loukopoulos *et al.* (2009) concluded that highly trained experts such as pilots are skilful at multitasking in their domains of expertise because they have extensive experience with the component tasks.

Another explanation often proposed for variation in multitasking performance is gender. Mäntylä (2013) explored this issue, concluding that her findings do not support the assumptions of a superior female capacity to handle multiple tasks. Outside research conditions, these results may appear distorted. The findings by Offer and Schneider (2011), that mothers spend 10 more hours a week multitasking compared with fathers and that these additional hours are mainly related to time spent on housework and childcare, may explain the discrepancy around these specific tasks.

In summary, it would appear for some activities that multitasking does not have a significant effect on performance whereas for others it can severely impair actions. This is dependent on the anatomical areas involved in the tasks and the current capacity and demands on the attentional system. It would seem that performance can be mediated by a practice effect whereby the attentional effort required is reduced through training.

Activity

Assess your own ability to do more than one thing at a time as follows. Perform at the same time:

- a verbal and a visual task, for example recite a poem or rhyme known by heart while doing a simple jigsaw
- two verbal tasks, for example listen to the radio while reading the newspaper.

Which is easier? Why?

Attention Systems

So far in this chapter, we have focused on different components of attention but we have also acknowledged that attention is a fundamental part of all cognitive function. Psychologists have been considering the role of attention in cognition since the end of the nineteenth century when William James distinguished between two modes of attention. The 'active' mode involves top-down processing related to a person's goals and expectations, and the 'passive' mode is reaction to external stimuli in a bottom-up way. Much of the research into attention since then has studied how we identify and respond to the stimuli in the external environment.

Attention Capacity

Early studies of attention processing (Kahneman 1973) described a capacity model with a central processor of limited capacity that flexibly allocates attention in parallel to the activities in progress (Figure 5.3). The total capacity of the central processor is affected by the level of arousal. Problems occur when the total demand of the tasks exceeds the attention capacity. Styles (1997) compared the capacity theory to a house with a limited gas supply. If the rings of the gas cooker are alight when the central heating boiler is activated, the jets on the cooker will go down. The demand of the two appliances together decreases the amount of gas available to the cooker. A rise in the pressure of the gas to the house would solve the problem of the cooker, in the same way that an increase in arousal has an effect on the total attention capacity.

The demands on attention capacity vary in several ways.

- *Mental effort* – novel and complex tasks demand a large share of the total attention capacity.
- *Skill* – the acquisition of skill at a task, as a result of practice, reduces the attention demands. Routine tasks that are familiar leave more capacity for an alternative activity.
- *Motivation and arousal* – higher levels increase the total capacity available for allocation. Performance increases with arousal up to an optimum.

Figure 5.3 Capacity model of attention. Source: Adapted from Kahneman (1973).

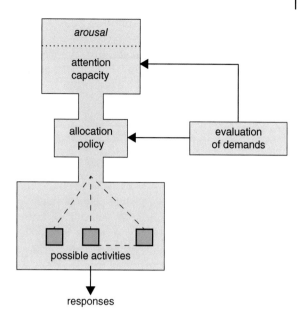

As previously illustrated, the capacity model does not fully account for the limitations of dividing attention between two activities, as these limitations are influenced by the anatomical proximity of the networks involved, and other factors. Developments of this model have replaced the single processor by multiple attention resources that are task specific.

The capacity model can explain the effects of brain damage when overall attention capacity is often reduced. Tasks that require high mental effort become too difficult, while tasks that were well known and familiar now become effortful. General arousal may also be reduced so that performance is slow and concentration is required in all activities. In this case, the environment needs to be controlled for the optimum performance of one task at a time. In contrast, the existence of 'multiple' processors can also be observed whereby some cognitive capacities can appear 'preserved' whereas others can demonstrate significant deficit.

Alerting, Orienting and Executive Attention Systems

Another theory is that attention consists of three highly connected yet independent networks (Posner and Petersen 1990) comprising alerting, orienting and executive attention systems (Posner and Rothbart 2007).

The alerting and orienting networks constitute the more primitive components of attention; the alerting system denotes sustained attention, vigilance or alertness, and refers to response readiness in preparation for an impending stimulus (Raz and Buhle 2006). This system may continue developing well into adulthood and is associated with the frontal and parietal regions of the right hemisphere (Marrocco and Davidson 1998). The more elaborate orienting network involves selecting specific information from multiple sensory stimuli (Raz and Buhle 2006) by mediating shifts of the sensory organs to bring objects of interest into focus (Posner and Rothbart 2007). It is associated with posterior brain areas, including the superior parietal lobe in addition to the frontal- eye fields (Gillen 2009), and is believed to develop fully by the age of four.

The complex executive system mediates voluntary control requiring the monitoring and resolution of conflict between competing attentional demands (Raz and Buhle 2006), such as in decision making or planning. It involves processes of self-regulation as well as inhibitory control, and is associated with the anterior cingulate and the lateral prefrontal cortex (Botvinick *et al.* 2001). This aspect of attention is dealt with in greater detail in Chapter 10.

Stimulus-Driven and Goal-Directed Attention

Posner and Peterson's description was later developed and extended by Corbetta and Shulman (2002) who described:

- a *stimulus-driven system* which detects salient stimuli in the environment and automatically shifts attention to them. This bottom-up system is activated when an important and unexpected stimulus is presented. Impairment of this system may explain why people with unilateral neglect ignore stimuli presented on the left side but they can voluntarily attend to that side (see Chapter 7)
- a *goal-directed system* controlled by the person's intentions, when the focus of attention is sustained on specific sensory information entering the brain. This top-down system is influenced by expectation, knowledge and goals. It overrides the automatic stimulus-driven system in the presence of confusing or competing elements in the environment. Impairment of this system leads to distractibility.

Brain imaging has provided a functional anatomy of the human attention system, and most researchers now conceive it as a system in which sequential processing occurs in stages using different brain networks (Lezak *et al.* 2004).

Impairments of Attention

In a review of the neuropsychological outcomes of stroke and its relationship to functional outcome, it was concluded that neuropsychological factors are more important determinants of functional outcomes after stroke than physical disability (Barker-Collo and Feigin 2006). This suggests that cognitive impairments are a greater determinant of rehabilitative outcomes and long-term disability than is often recognised.

Not only do cognitive impairments potentially determine rehabilitation outcomes but there are a significant number of people experiencing attentional problems, as a result of a variety of different neurological conditions.

Hochstenbach *et al.* (1998) studied neuropsychological functioning in 229 individuals assessed two months post stroke and found that over 70% suffered impaired information processing. The same researchers discovered that attention deficits improved on average by between only 7% and 28% (depending on the locus of the lesion) at a two-year follow-up. Similar results were found by Leśniak *et al.* (2008), who assessed the cognition of 200 consecutive patients two weeks after their first stroke and re-examined 80 of them a year later. Seventy-eight per cent of patients were found to be impaired in one or more cognitive domains at the postacute stage, with attention being the most common deficit (48.5%). On follow-up, attention deficits were still found to be the most frequent symptom.

Improvements in attention have been found to occur in the weeks following stroke and the estimated frequency of the deficit over time lies between 46–92% on discharge and 20–43% four years later (Hyndman and Ashburn 2003; Stapleton *et al.* 2001). The wide range reported may reflect the different types of attentional deficits under consideration.

In people with multiple sclerosis, Nocentini *et al.* (2006) reported cognitive dysfunction, including attentional deficits, in 40–60% of individuals with the relapsing-remitting type. A study of elderly people concluded that dementia is a considerable health problem in the population aged between 75 and 80 years old (de Deyn *et al.* 2011), a health condition in which difficulties with attention and alertness are common. Finally, in children, the prevalence of attention deficit hyperactivity disorder (ADHD) in the UK is estimated to be between 0.5% and 1.5%, although it has been suggested that this is an underestimation due to difficulties with diagnostic criteria (Graham *et al.* 2007).

Effect on Function

When considering the functional consequences of attentional deficits, it is interesting to note the conclusion of Robertson *et al.* (1997) that sustained attention is predictive of both functional status two years post stroke and outcomes from rehabilitation. These assertions suggest that the presence of attentional deficits should inform both predictions of progress from rehabilitation and the long-term functioning of an individual, such as their ability to live independently or to return to work and social activity (Leśniak *et al.* 2008; Paolucci *et al.* 1996). More specifically, studies have discovered associations between distractibility, auditory selective attention, balance and functional impairment among acute stroke patients (Stapleton *et al.* 2001). Similar findings were reported between ability in activities of daily living, balance and sustained and divided attention in community-dwelling people with stroke (Hyndman and Ashburn 2003). This may explain those individuals who persist in falling despite no obvious findings of physical or mechanical difficulties (de Bruin and Schmidt 2010).

Attentional deficits can limit a person's ability to learn and retain information, can impair ability to monitor the environment and make appropriate responses, to maintain focus on and complete tasks or to discriminate relevant from irrelevant sensory information. These all have implications for safety, independence and progress in rehabilitation.

Factors Influencing Attention

As previously suggested, attention is dependent on both internal and external factors and as such has been associated with a number of impairments. Those that have been found to have a direct influence on attention, and therefore need to be addressed within any treatment programme, include anxiety and emotions (Lystad *et al.* 2009), subjective fatigue and disturbed sleep (Zerouali *et al.* 2010; Ziino and Ponsford 2006), exercise (Aks 1998) and also (in animal studies) the environment (Maffei 2012).

The box below contains an edited description of an individual's experience of living with attentional deficits. Specifically, the contributor has (as he describes) attention deficit disorder (ADD) and therefore it is difficult to generalise this to other acquired conditions, such as brain injury. However, it provides a taste of both the positive and negative aspects of the condition.

The lived experience of attentional deficits (Hallowell 2012)

ADD is like driving in the rain with bad windshield wipers. Everything smudges and blurs and you speed along. It's reeeeally frustrating not being able to see clearly. Or, it's like listening to the radio with lots of static and you have to strain to hear what's going on. In ADD, time collapses into a black hole. It feels like everything happens all at once. There's a sense of inner turmoil, you lose perspective and cannot prioritise. You're always on the go, trying to keep the world from caving in. You feel you are being pulled invisibly in all directions, and people label you disorganised and impulsive.

I can't keep still. I fidget, scratch, doodle so people think I'm uninterested or not paying attention. My wife has learned not to take my tuning out personally – she says that when I'm there, I'm really there.

The thing about ADD is that it takes lots of adapting and time to get on in life. However, there is a positive side. Often people with ADD are highly imaginative and intuitive. They have a 'feel' for situations, and can see right into the heart of matters unlike the methodical reasoning of others. Their cognitive style is qualitatively different from most people. What may seem impaired can, with patience and encouragement, become gifted.

The good news is that treatment can really help. Learning to structure one's life, exercise programmes, small spurts of activity, breaking down tasks into smaller tasks, support groups, medication – these all help to turn down the noise.

Suggestions for Assessment and Intervention

The Society for Cognitive Rehabilitation (2008) has recommended the early identification and rehabilitation of attention deficits.

Assessment

- Assessments of attention need to be varied and repeated during different activities and under diverse conditions because attention is variable and context dependent.
- Assessments of impairment are usually standardised with a level of established validity and reliability (see Table 5.1 for examples). They are often unable to predict performance in specific activities and environments and so are insufficient to use on their own.
- The Assessment of Motor and Process Skills (AMPS) (Fischer 2003) is an observational assessment of occupational performance against 16 motor and 20 process skill items. This assessment enables an understanding of ability at the activity level.
- Assessment of environment is generally carried out informally whereby individuals are exposed to more varied and demanding environments to identify their attentional capacity and any environmental factors mediating attention, and also to evaluate the use of compensatory strategies. These observations should ideally include the pertinent physical, social and attitudinal factors within the environment (WHO 2001).

Table 5.1 Selected assessments of attention and ICF domains.

Assessment tool	Description	ICF dimension measured
QBTest Plus (Lis *et al.* 2010)	ADHD specific: combines computerised continuous performance tests with the measurement of motor activity	Body functions tested via simulated activities Simultaneous recording of motor activity
Attention Rating and Monitoring Scale (Cicerone 2002)	Self-report of the frequency of problems attributable to attentional impairments	Body functions identified during everyday observation
Test of Everyday Attention (Robertson *et al.* 1996)	Considered an ecologically valid test of various types of everyday attention	Body functions tested via simulated activities
Wessex Head Injury Matrix (WHIM) (Shiel *et al.* 2000)	Behavioural scale to assess and monitor recovery after severe brain injury. Specific attentional deficits included in the 62 items	Impairments across six areas: communication; attention; social behaviour; concentration; visual awareness; cognition
Test of Everyday Attention for Children (Anderson *et al.* 1998)	Considered an ecologically valid test of various types of everyday attention	Body functions tested via simulated activities
Moss Attention Rating Scale for Traumatic Brain Injury (Whyte *et al.* 2003)	Structural observation of basic activities to identify underlying attentional deficits	Body functions and activity domains

Intervention

Consider education, process training (remediation), strategy development and implementation (compensation) and functional application.

- *Remediation* – a number of studies have evaluated the effectiveness of the frequently used Attention Process Training (APT), identifying an effect at the impairment level, but with insufficient evidence of carryover into everyday activities (Barker-Collo *et al.* 2009; Bowman *et al.* 2004; Park *et al.* 1999). Other diverse interventions that have been evaluated as mediating attention include mindfulness training (Chiesa *et al.* 2011), singing (Helding 2012) and interacting with nature (Berman *et al.* 2008).
- *Compensation* – included in this approach are methods such as psychological adaptation (to enable the individual to accommodate for their disability as opposed to focusing exclusively on remediation of their deficits), reduction in competing attentional demands within the chosen activity, addressing those factors directly associated with the individual's attentional problems and modification of the environment to reduce distraction. A review evaluating the current evidence for these approaches concluded that rehabilitation is effective in helping patients learn and apply compensations for residual cognitive limitations, although several studies suggest that intervention may directly improve underlying cognitive functions (Cicerone *et al.* 2011).

SUMMARY

1) Attention has a significant influence on performance as it has been described as 'the underlying foundation for all other cognitive skills' and is considered 'the prerequisite condition upon which the dynamic dance between memory and learning depends'.
2) Neurophysiological arousal is necessary for attention. Too little or too much arousal can adversely impact upon performance, rendering a person incapable of attending at all, or unable to direct and control his or her own attentional resources appropriately.
3) Attention is classified into different functional types: selective, sustained, alternating or shifting, and divided (also known as multitasking).
4) Attentional capacity is a limited resource, and stimuli can make competing demands upon it. Activities make different levels and types of demand depending upon the amount of mental effort required, the sensory modalities being used (same or different), the person's level of skill or familiarity with the task, environmental conditions and the person's level of motivation and arousal. Capacity can be exceeded. Models of attention variously posit capacity and sequential processing in separate but related networks as key features.
5) Evidence indicates that there is a high prevalence of attentional deficits across a number of different health conditions and that they often persevere. These difficulties are frequently masked until an individual is required to engage in complex or novel activities and therefore go unacknowledged, despite their profound effect on rehabilitation and functional outcomes. This situation is further confused by the different types of attention, the number of factors that directly influence it and the fluctuating nature of the problem.
6) There is evidence to suggest that both remediative and compensatory interventions may have positive effects upon attention.

References

Aks, D. (1998) Influence of exercise on visual search: implications for mediating cognitive mechanisms. *Perceptual and Motor Skills*, **87**, 771–783.

Allport, D.A., Antonis, B. and Reynolds, P. (1972) On the division of attention: a disproof of the single channel hypothesis. *Quarterly Journal of Experimental Psychology*, **24**, 225–235.

Amos, A. (2002) Remediating deficits of switching attention in patients with acquired brain injury. *Brain Injury*, **16** (5), 407–413.

Anderson, V., Fenwick, T., Manley, T. and Robertson, I. (1998) Attentional skills following traumatic brain injury in childhood: a componential analysis. *Brain Injury*, **12** (11), 937–949.

Barker-Collo, S. and Feigin, V. (2006) The impact of neurospsychological deficits on functional stroke outcomes. *Neuropsychology Review*, **16**, 53–64.

Barker-Collo, S.L., Feigin, V.L., Lawes, C.M., Parag, V., Senior, H. and Rodgers, A. (2009) Reducing attention deficits after stroke using attention process training: a randomized controlled trial. *STROKE*, **40** (10), 3293–3298.

Beck, D.M. and Kastner, S. (2007) Stimulus similarity modulates competitive interactions in human visual cortex. *Journal of Vision*, **7** (2), 19.1–12.

Berman, M.G., Jonides, J. and Kaplan, S. (2008) The cognitive benefits of interacting with nature. *Psychological Science*, **19** (12), 1207–1212.

Boman, I., Lindsted, M., Hemmingsson, H. and Bartfai, A. (2004) Cognitive training in home environment. *Brain Injury*, **18** (10), 985–995.

Botvinick, M.M., Braver, T.S., Barch, D.M., Carter, C.S and Cohen, J.D. (2001) Conflict monitoring and cognitive control. *Psychological Review*, **108** (3), 624–652.

Broadbent, D. (1958) *Perception and Communication*, Pergamon Press, London.

Bruin, E. and Schmidt, A. (2010) Walking behaviour of healthy elderly: attention should be paid. *Behavioral and Brain Functions*, **6**, 59. Available at: www.behavioralandbrainfunctions.com/content/6/1/59 (accessed 22 September 2016).

Carrasco, M. (2011) Visual attention: the past 25 years. *Vision Research*, **51** (13), 1484–1525.

Cicerone, K. (2002) Remediation of 'working attention' in mild traumatic brain injury. *Brain Injury*, **16** (13), 185–195.

Cicerone, K.D., Langenbahn, D.M., Braden, C. *et al.* (2011) Evidence-based cognitive rehabilitation: updated review of the literature from 2003 through 2008 *Archives of Physical Medicine and Rehabilitation*, **92** (4), 519–530.

Chiesa, A., Calati, R. and Serretti, A. (2011) Does mindfulness training improve cognitive abilities? A systematic review of neuropsychological findings. *Clinical Psychology Review*, **31**, 449–464.

Corbetta, M. and Shulman, G.L. (2002) Control of goal-directed and stimulus-driven attention in the brain. *Nature Reviews Neuroscience*, **3** (3), 201–215.

De Deyn, P.P., Goeman, J., Vervaet, A., Dourcy-Belle-Rose, B., van Dam, D. and Geerts, E. (2011) Prevalence and incidence of dementia among 75–80-year-old community-dwelling elderly in different districts of Antwerp, Belgium: the Antwerp Cognition (ANCOG) Study. *Clinical Neurology and Neurosurgery*, **113**, 736–745.

Desimone, R. and Duncan, J. (1995) Neural mechanisms of selective visual attention. *Annual Review of Neuroscience*, **18**,193–222.

Drews, F.A., Pasupathi, M. and Strayer, D.L. (2008) Passenger and cell-phone conversations in simulated driving. *Journal of Experimental Psychology: Applied*, **14**, 392–400.

Drews, F., Yazdani, H., Godfrey, C., Cooper, J. and Strayer, L. (2009) Text messaging during simulated driving. *Human Factors*, **51** (5), 762–770.

Fischer, A. (2003) *Assessment of Motor and Process Skills, Vol 1: Development, Standardisation and Administration Manual*, 5th edn, Three Star Press, Fort Collins, Colorado.

Gillen, G. (2009) *Cognitive and Perceptual Rehabilitation. Optimizing Function*, Mosby Elsevier, St Louis, Missouri.

Graham, J., Seth, S. and Coghill, D. (2007) What's new in … ADHD. *Medicine*, **35** (3), 181–185.

Hallowell, E.M. (2012) What's it like to have ADHD? http://www.drhallowell.com/whats-it-like-to-have-adhd (accessed 14 December 2016).

Helding, L. (2012) Choosing attention. *Journal of Singing*, **68** (3), 321–327.

Hochstenbach, J., Mulder, T., van Limbeek, J., Donders, R. and Schoonderwaldt, H. (1998) Cognitive decline following stroke: a comprehensive study of cognitive decline following stroke. *Journal of Clinical and Experimental Neuropsychology*, **20** (4), 503–517.

Hyndman, D. and Ashburn, A. (2003) People with stroke living in the community: attention deficits, balance, ADL ability and falls. *Disability and Rehabilitation*, **25**, 817–822.

Kahneman, D. (1973) *Attention and Effort*, Prentice Hall, Englewood Cliffs, New Jersey.

Kastner, S. and Ungerleider, L. (2000) Mechanisms of visual attention in the human cortex. *Annual Review of Neuroscience*, **23**, 315–341.

Kastner, S., de Weerd, P., Desimone, R. and Ungerleider, L.G. (1998) Mechanisms of directed attention in the human extrastriate cortex as revealed by functional MRI. *Science*, **282**, 108–111.

Kinchla, R.A. (1992) Attention. *Annual Review of Psychology*, **43**, 711–742.

Kinsbourne, M. and Hicks, R.E. (1978) Functional cerebral space: a model for overflow, transfer and interference effects in human performance: a tutorial review, in *Attention and Performance VII* (ed. J. Requin), Erlbaum, Hillsdale, New Jersey, pp. 345–362.

Leclercq, M. (2002) Theoretical aspects of the main components and functions of attention, in *Applied Neuropsychology of Attention: Theory, Diagnosis and Rehabilitation* (eds M. Leclercq and P. Zimmermann), Psychology Press, New York, pp. 3–55.

Leśniak, M., Bak, T., Czepiel, W., Seniów, J. and Członkowska, A. (2008) Frequency and prognostic value of cognitive disorders in stroke patients. *Dementia and Geriatric Cognitive Disorders*, **26**, 356–363.

Lezak, M., Howieson, D. and Loring, D. (2004) *Neuropsychological Assessment*, 4th edn, Oxford University Press, New York.

Lis, S., Baer, N., Stein-en-Nosse, C., Gallhofer, B., Sammer, G. and Kirsch, P. (2010) Objective measurement of motor activity during cognitive performance in adults with attention deficit/hyperactivity disorder. *Acta Psychiatrica Scandinavica*, **122**, 285–294.

Loukopoulos, L.D., Dismukes, R.K. and Barshi, I. (2009) *The Multitasking myth: Handling Complexity in Real-World Operations*, Ashgate, Farnham.

Lystad, C.M., Rokke, P.D. and Stout, D.M. (2009) Emotion congruent facilitation of attention when processing anxious stimuli. *Cognitive Therapy and Research*, **33** (5), 499–510.

Maffei, A. (2012) Enriching the environment to disinhibit the brain and improve cognition. *Frontiers in Cellular Neuroscience*, **6** (53). Available at: www.ncbi.nlm.nih.gov/pmc/articles/PMC3498904/ (accessed 22 September 2016).

Mäntylä, T. (2013) Gender differences in multitasking reflect spatial ability. *Psychological Science*, **24** (4), 514–520.

Marrocco, R. and Davidson, M. (1998) *Neurochemistry of attention, in The Attentive Brain Vol. XII* (ed. R. Parasuraman), MIT Press, Cambridge, Massachusetts, pp. 35–50.

Nocentini, U., Pasqualetti, P., Bonavita, S. *et al.* (2006) Cognitive dysfunction in patients with relapsing-remitting multiple sclerosis. *Multiple Sclerosis*, **12**, 77–87.

Offer, S. and Schneider, B. (2011) Revisiting the gender gap in time use patterns: multitasking and well-being among mothers and fathers in dual-earner families. *American Sociological Review*, **76**, 809–833.

Paolucci, S., Antonucci, G., Gialloretti, L. *et al.* (1996) Predicting stroke inpatient rehabilitation outcome: the predominant role of neuropsychological disorders. *European Neurology*, **36**, 385–390.

Park, N.W., Proulx, G. and Towers, W.M. (1999) Evaluation of the attention process training programme. *Neuropsychological Rehabilitation*, **9** (2), 135–154.

Penner, I. and Kappos, L. (2006) Retraining attention in MS. *Journal of the Neurological Sciences*, **245** (1–2), 147–151.

Posner, M.I. and Petersen, S.E. (1990) The attention system of the human brain. *Annual Review of Neuroscience*, **13**, 25–42.

Posner, M.I. and Rothbart, M.K. (2007) Research on attention networks as a model for the integration of psychological science. *Annual Review of Psychology*, **58**, 1–23.

Raz, A. and Buhle, J. (2006) Typologies of attentional networks. *Nature Reviews Neuroscience*, **7** (5), 367–379.

Ries, M. and Marks, W. (2005) Selective attention deficits following severe closed head injury: the role of inhibitory processes. *Neuropsychology*, **19** (4), 476–483.

Robertson, I.H., Ward, T., Ridgeway, V. and Nimmo-Smith, I. (1996) The structure of normal human attention: the test of everyday attention. *Journal of Clinical and Experimental Neuropsychology*, **2** (6), 525–534.

Robertson, I.H., Ridgeway, V., Greenfield, E. and Parr, A. (1997) Motor recovery after stroke depends on intact sustained attention: a 2-year follow-up study. *Neuropsychology*, **11**, 290–295.

Shiel, A., Horn, S., Wilson, B., Watson, M., Campbell, M. and Mclellan, D. (2000) The Wessex Head Injury Matrix (WHIM) main scale: a preliminary report on a scale to assess and monitor patient recovery after severe head injury. *Clinical Rehabilitation*, **14**, 408–416.

Society for Cognitive Rehabilitation Guidelines (2008) *Recommendations for Best Practice in Cognitive Rehabilitation Therapy: Acquired Brain Injury*. Available at: www.societyforcognitiverehab.org/membership-and-certification/documents/EditedRecsBestPrac.pdf (accessed 22 September 2016).

Sohlberg, M.M. and Mateer, C.A. (2001) *Cognitive Rehabilitation: An Integrative Neuropsychological Approach*, Guilford Press, New York.

Spelke, E., Hirst, W. and Neisser, U. (1976) Skills of divided attention. *Cognition*, **4**, 215–230.

Stapleton, T., Ashburn, A. and Stack, E. (2001) A pilot study of attention deficits, balance control and falls in the subacute stage following stroke. *Clinical Rehabilitation*, **15**, 437–444.

Strayer, D.L., Drews, F.A. and Johnston, W.A. (2003) Cell phone induced failures of visual attention during simulated driving. *Journal of Experimental Psychology: Applied*, **9**, 23–52.

Styles, E.A. (1997) *The Psychology of Attention*, Psychology Press, Hove.

Treisman, A.M. and Gelade, G. (1980) A feature-integration theory of attention. *Cognitive Psychology*, **12**, 97–136.

Whyte, J. (1992) Attention and arousal: basic science aspects. *Archives of Physical Medicine and Rehabilitation*, **10**, 940–949.

Whyte, J., Hart, T., Bode, R.K. and Malec, J.F. (2003) The Moss Attention Rating Scale for traumatic brain injury: initial psychometric assessment. *Archives of Physical Medicine and Rehabilitation*, **84** (2), 268–276.

World Health Organisation (2001) *The International Classification of Functioning, Disability and Health*, World Health Organisation, Geneva.

Zerouali, Y., Jemel, B. and Godbout, R. (2010) The effects of early and late night partial sleep deprivation on automatic and selective attention: an ERP study. *Brain Research*, **1308**, 87–99.

Ziino, C. and Ponsford, J. (2006) Selective attention deficits and subjective fatigue following traumatic brain injury. *Neuropsychology*, **20** (3), 383–390.

6

Visual Perception, Recognition and Agnosia

Linda Maskill and June Grieve

AIMS

1) To provide an outline of basic visual functions and the sensory processing of visual information.
2) To introduce the basic components of visual perceptual processing and object recognition.
3) To appreciate the nature and importance of perception in other sensory modalities, and their contribution to functional independence.
4) To gain understanding of visual and tactile agnosia, and their functional implications.
5) To consider approaches, methods and tools for assessment and intervention for visual and tactile agnosia.

Introduction

Visual perception gives meaning to all the information entering the eyes. Vision plays a major role in the total perception of the environment and the brain has a larger area of cerebral cortex devoted to the processing of vision than any of the other senses. In the constantly changing visual environment, we perceive individual objects, people and landmarks as the same, whatever their position, illumination or distance from us.

The adaptability of visual perception was dramatically illustrated in an experiment when subjects wore spectacles with inverting lenses. After several days, the subjects had adapted to the upside-down view of the world. They were able to move around normally and perform all daily living activities. Our ability to instantly recognise the features of the visual environment seems to be so easy that it is difficult to appreciate how many complex processes are involved. To represent a scene in drawing or painting, we have to think about size, depth, distance, light and shade. The great landscape painters in the early nineteenth century were the pioneers for the representation of these features on a flat canvas. The Impressionist painters were able to create three-dimensional scenes using flat planes of colour.

Neuropsychology for Occupational Therapists: Cognition in Occupational Performance, Fourth Edition.
Edited by Linda Maskill and Stephanie Tempest.
© 2017 John Wiley & Sons Ltd. Published 2017 by John Wiley & Sons Ltd.
Companion Website: www.wiley.com/go/maskill/neuropsychologyOT

Looking around a room, each object is isolated from its background, and from other objects adjacent to it. As we look out of the window, we can decide where a house ends and a tree begins, if they are overlapping. When we move about, landmarks are recognised and obstructions are avoided. The recognition of objects is associated with meaning and function for their use. In social interaction, we recognise faces and associate them with the names of the people we know. Complex cognitive processing is involved to convert the retinal image into our perception of the three-dimensional world.

The person with visual perceptual deficits functions below the expected level but is often unaware of any problem. When objects are only partially exposed to view, or are seen from unusual angles, there is difficulty in recognising them. Poor object recognition leads to problems with daily living tasks, particularly when several objects are used. In some cases it is possible to recognise objects from touch or from a verbal description. Face recognition problems affect the ability to communicate with others, leading to isolation and loss of independence. The basic visual functions of visual acuity and co-ordination of eye movements, as well as a deficit in visual perception, may be underlying factors in the impairment of any component of cognition.

Basic Visual Functions

The processing of depth, orientation and motion forms the basis of visuospatial perception. These must be supported by the basic visual functions:

- visual acuity
- visual field and
- eye movement control.

Cate and Richards (2000) emphasised the importance of these functions in a bottom-up approach for the evaluation of higher level visuospatial skills. Sand *et al.* (2013) described the impact of disorders of basic visual functions upon recovery of independence following stroke, identifying their critical role and the importance of detecting and addressing such deficits in rehabilitation.

Visual Acuity

Visual acuity is the ability to see small detail at all distances from the eyes. It is measured using high-contrast letter charts. Acuity also depends on contrast sensitivity, which is the ability to detect the borders of objects by contrast from their backgrounds. Loss of contrast sensitivity makes reading words on a page difficult. This occurs with normal ageing and can be improved by increasing illumination.

Loss of visual acuity is common in older people and may exacerbate the impact of other impairments, for example postural instability leading to an increased risk of falls or neurological disorders such as stroke that give rise to impairments of visuospatial perception. Often, people may not have kept up with regular eye examinations, and have glasses with outdated prescription lenses. In a study of 77 older people admitted to a hospital for rehabilitation following stroke, Lotery *et al.* (2000) found that 25% did not have their glasses with them, and 23% had glasses that were unacceptably dirty, scratched or damaged. Eleven patients experienced an improvement in visual acuity when their glasses prescriptions were updated.

Figure 6.1 Visual field and the visual pathway. Information from one visual field enters both eyes and projects to the visual cortex of the opposite hemisphere.

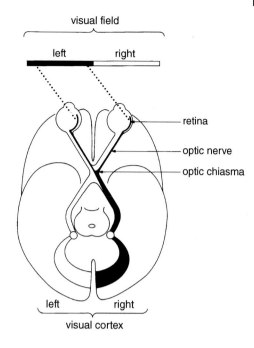

Visual Field

The visual field is the area of view of the external world seen by the two eyes without movement of the head. The visual field is like a window to the visual world. The view through the window can be scanned by movements of the eyes. Movements of the head take the window to different positions around the scene and this increases the area that can be scanned. The visual fields for the right and left eyes overlap in the midline, so that some light from each visual field reaches the retina of both eyes.

The visual pathway from one half of the visual field for each eye reaches the occipital lobe of the opposite side. In Figure 6.1, follow the projection from the left visual field to the inner nasal half of the left retina, and to the outer temporal half of the right retina. Now continue the same path (shown in black) on to the optic chiasma and then to the right occipital lobe. There is a mapping of the visual field in the primary visual cortex V1 around the calcarine sulcus. You should now appreciate how damage to the right primary visual cortex V1 in the occipital lobe produces 'blind areas' in the left visual field.

The following activities demonstrate how the area of the normal visual field can be estimated simply and the experience of the loss of a part of the visual field in both eyes.

Activity

- Stand behind a partner and ask him/her to focus on an object straight ahead. Place your fingers at different positions in the subject's visual field ahead – to either side, above and below. Ask your partner to report when the fingers are seen.
- Cut out quarters or halves of a circle in black paper. Stick pairs of corresponding shapes on to the inner half of one lens and the outer half of the other lens of a pair of spectacles. Wear the spectacles while you walk about, write, read and make a cup of coffee. Ask someone to observe your compensatory head movements.

The loss of half the visual field is known as hemianopia. If the lesion is restricted to one bank of the calcarine sulcus in V1, there is loss of vision in one-quarter of the visual field, known as quadrantanopia. Damage above the calcarine sulcus leads to a blind area in a lower quadrant, while damage below the calcarine sulcus results in a blind area in an upper quadrant of the visual field.

Small areas of cell necrosis or damage in the primary visual cortex V1 around the calcarine sulcus produce small patches of blind areas in the visual field. These scomata often occur in traumatic brain injury. Some people with scomata are unaware of the problem if visual perception fills in the blind areas. Loss of the central area of the visual field, associated with demyelination of the optic nerve, occurs in multiple sclerosis. Diplopia (double vision) reduces the ability to discriminate form. All these changes in basic visual function affect spatial perception.

A person with a visual field defect does not see objects clearly. Many people develop strategies to overcome the partial loss of vision but even with compensation strategies, reading often remains a problem. In scanning the page from left to right, the person with loss of the right visual field cannot make sense of the text after the first few words. The person with a left visual field defect cannot start to read, or has difficulty in picking up the next line as the eyes return to the left. People with unilateral neglect have similar problems with reading but they are able to read the words when the head is turned (see Chapter 7).

Case study (Andrewes 2001)

CG suffered a cerebral haemorrhage which resulted in quadrantanopia in the lower left half of his vision. He reported that his vision seemed fuzzy and dim in parts. When he looked ahead, his vision became darker or dimmer. If he looked around, the dark left lower area interfered with the rest of his vision and everything became somehow less clear. The compensation strategy he developed was to look steadily to the left. He could not drive because cars popped up from nowhere on the left side. He was unable to see clearly enough to cut up food and could not read properly. He developed a strategy of looking steadily to the left to compensate.

Eye Movements

The ability to scan the space around us depends on the control of eye movements by the oculomotor system in the brainstem, together with movements of the head. Other oculomotor functions are to maintain binocular vision, fixate on a target ahead, follow moving targets and maintain a stable gaze when the head moves. The extraocular muscles, which execute the movements of the eyes, are innervated by three cranial nerves originating in the brainstem. Projections from the occipital and frontal cortex to the nuclei of these nerves in the brainstem form a system for the control of eye movements. A stable gaze is maintained by input from the vestibular system which responds to movements of the head.

Two different types of eye movement occur in following a moving image and in scanning a static display.

- A *pursuit eye movement* is a slow movement of the eyes at the same rate as a moving image in order to keep the image on the central part of the retina. They only occur when the eye is tracking a moving target. Pursuit movements of the eyes originate in the occipital lobes.
- *Saccadic eye movements* are made in scanning a static display. They are used to quickly direct the gaze towards an object of interest. The eyes fixate on the item, for example a group of words on a page, and then make a rapid eye movement or saccade to the next item. In scanning a larger area such as a picture, the eyes first make long saccades from the centre to the periphery, followed by shorter and shorter saccades to fixate on the detail of the picture. Saccadic movements of the eyes originate in the supplementary motor area of the frontal lobes. This area activates the brainstem nuclei of the extraocular muscles to produce a rapid movement of the eyes to the opposite side.

Activity

1) Ask a partner to fixate on the tip of a pencil while you move it across from left to right. Observe how the eyes move slowly as they follow the target. This is a pursuit eye movement.
2) Ask a partner to move his/her eyes in a straight line from left to right. You will see the eyes make alternating fixation and rapid saccades as they scan the path from left to right.
3) Use a small coloured ball at the end of a black wand. Ask a partner to:
   - follow the ball as you move it slowly in different directions – up and down, from left to right, and from right to left
   - fixate on the ball held in one position.

A person with problems in scanning cannot keep their eyes on the ball.

Pursuit eye movements are used to track objects as we move them around in functional activity and to follow the course of a moving vehicle along the road. These tracking eye movements are used in sports activities and in computer games when the eyes must follow a ball or a figure as it moves towards a target. We make saccadic eye movements across the words on a page in reading. Saccades also occur when we view successive landmarks in travel on a bus or a train. The ability to maintain a stable gaze is important when the whole body moves in space. The head moves with each step in walking but the eyes keep a stable gaze ahead.

Disruption of the oculomotor system leads to slower speed of eye movements and poor visual scanning. After traumatic brain injury, the eye movements are often spontaneous and erratic. Random scanning movements lead to delay in interpreting an image. Loss of co-ordination of the movements of both eyes to focus on a target may lead to double vision and poor depth perception. Poor saccadic eye movements make reading difficult.

Early Visual Processing

The retina of each eye receives a two-dimensional image of the visual field ahead. The role of visual perception is to convert this constantly changing image into a three-dimensional object or scene which has meaning. The features which form the perceptual analysis of the environment are colour, shape, size, depth, figure ground and motion. Early screening for shape and colour can be done with a form board. The brain-damaged person is asked to fit coloured wooden shapes of different forms into corresponding shapes on the board.

Sensory information about surface texture and the direction of lines and edges also contributes to visual perception. Outlines of landmarks are isolated from their background. Perceptions of objects are stable even when they are seen in different views.

Colour

Colour in the visual environment gives added meaning. Colour perception is different from colour blindness, which is a retinal defect. In child development, the toddler learns that the colour and form of particular objects are associated with their function. Even in different lighting conditions, familiar objects do not change their colour. Similar items that can be present in different colours, for example coins or food in jars, depend on colour discrimination for identification. When there is loss of colour perception, the world is seen as shades of grey, and vision is reported as 'not clear' even though visual acuity is normal. Loss of colour can occur in one-half of the visual field. A photograph of a bunch of flowers is then seen as one half in colour and the other half in white.

Selective impairment of colour and shape has been described in some people with cerebral damage. This suggests that in early visual processing, colour is processed separately from shape.

The inability to recognise colour, in the absence of retinal defects, is known as *achromatopsia* or colour agnosia. The person with colour agnosia is unable to match colours or sort different shades of the same colour. In a severe form which occurs in bilateral posterior lesions, the visual environment is seen as black, white or grey. Some loss of colour discrimination, particularly in the blue end of the spectrum, is common in cerebral lesions. An apparent loss of colour perception in the person with right hemiplegia is more likely to be due to a colour naming problem.

If colour perception is impaired, faces and common objects can usually be recognised from other features, but problems arise in the use of money when bronze and silver coins appear the same. In sorting out clothes, the person relies on tactile cues and cannot colour match or co-ordinate separate items. There is difficulty in distinguishing foods in jars, and in the selection of items such as tins of soup or beans from a shelf in the supermarket. Mistakes are often only realised from the smell and taste of food when the tin is opened.

Figure Ground

In the 1920s, the Gestalt psychologists first proposed that perception is organised to produce 'good form'. They introduced the term figure ground. In the visual world, we perceive whole objects set in a background. All the items and objects we use must be

Figure 6.2 Perception of depth and figure ground.

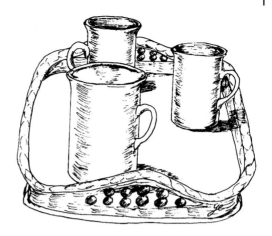

isolated from the surfaces they are on and from other objects that overlap them. The three mugs shown in Figure 6.2 are the 'figure' and the tray is the 'ground'.

Activity
Look around the room you are in and count the number of objects you can see. Then count how many of the objects are overlapped by other objects. Move to the other side of the room where you see different views of the same objects and at different distances. Note the shadows cast by the light from the window or lamp falling on the objects, and how the textures of surfaces change in the distance. All these features contribute to visual perception of the environment.

Visual perception segments the environment into what is figure and what is ground. It is the grouping together of the elements of colour, form and depth that produces the figure and separates it from the ground. Many visual illusions are pictures where the figure and the ground can be exchanged. Figure 6.3 can be perceived as a vase or two faces in silhouette, depending on whether the black area or the white area is coded in the brain as the ground, respectively.

A person with impairment of figure ground has difficulty in picking out objects when they are surrounded by others, for example a fork in a drawer of cutlery. The person cannot find things, for example the soap in the bathroom, a comb in a drawer or a cup in a cupboard. In dressing, items of clothing cannot be isolated from the bedcover they are lying on, especially a white T-shirt lying on a white sheet.

Depth perception comes partly from the difference in the image of an object received by the brain from the retina of each eye. There are, however, other clues in the visual field which provide information about depth. If one object partly obscures another, the complete object is perceived to be nearer. When similar objects appear to be different sizes, the larger ones are perceived to be nearer and the smaller ones further away. Parallel lines appear to converge and textures become finer in the distance. The mugs on a tray in Figure 6.2 illustrate these clues to depth perception.

The perception of depth is basic to constructional ability and finding our way around (see Chapter 7). Movement in the environment gives clues about depth. When sitting in

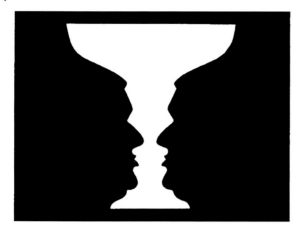

Figure 6.3 Figure ground – two different interpretations.

a moving car, nearby features of the visual scene, such as telegraph poles, appear to move by quickly while distant trees appear to move slowly.

Perceptual Constancy

Perceptual constancy is the feature of visual perception that allows us to recognise shapes and objects as the same when presented in a variety of conditions. Size discrimination is part of form constancy. We can distinguish the same shape seen in different sizes from other shapes or objects. My table appears the same size when I stand 1 metre away or 6 metres across the room. As I move about the room, I do not see the table moving about, even though the image of the table on my retina is changing. If I tilt my head to one side, the retinal image again changes but the table appears the same. When we view the same object in different size, orientation or brightness, the retinal image is different but we recognise the object as the same (Figure 6.4). If we are shown an unfamiliar object, we can still identify it as the same object when we see it from above, from below, at an angle, and so on. This is known as perceptual constancy and without it, the visual world would be very confusing.

Perceptual constancy may be explained by the additional information provided in the background context. Optical illusions occur when the context triggers inaccurate perceptual constancy.

People with deficits in form constancy have difficulty in recognising familiar items or objects when they appear in unusual orientation and without a background. There may be problems in kitchen tasks in selecting the appropriate item and using it correctly. In dressing, a garment may not be recognised if it is upside down or inside out.

Motion

Visual perception includes the interpretation of movement occurring in the environment. Movement separates items from their background. It may be easier to recognise a person in a crowd if he or she is moving. We observe wind direction from the moving trees.

Figure 6.4 Object constancy.

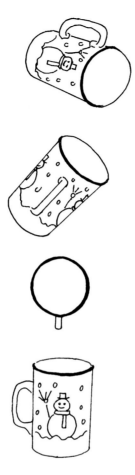

The direction of movement of a bus is known from the sequence of images projected on to the retina. We can estimate the speed of traffic from the movement of vehicles along the road. This perceptual processing of motion is an important part of our total visual perception.

Case study (Zihl *et al.* 1983)

A case was reported of a woman who had selective impairment of motion perception. MP had brain damage revealed in a CT scan as bilateral lesions in the temporal lobe and parietotemporal junction. She was able to match for colour and shape, and had normal tactile and auditory perception but she experienced selective loss of motion perception, particularly stimuli moving at high speeds. Movement was perceived as a series of static snapshots with moving objects appearing in one position and then another. The tea she poured into a cup appeared to her like a glacier and she failed to notice when it was overflowing. Unable to cross the road safely, she became confined to her home and was misdiagnosed as agoraphobic.

No similar severe cases have been reported but it has been shown that transcranial magnetic stimulation (TMS) over the visual cortex can affect the ability to judge whether a stimulus moves to the left or right. This condition of *akinetopsia* may only occur in bilateral lesions. Case studies of the impairment of colour perception without loss of motion perception have been reported. Therefore the case study described above supports a double dissociation and evidence for separable processing of colour and motion.

In summary, the perception of colour, shape, figure ground, depth, motion and perceptual constancy form the early bottom-up processing which interacts with top-down processing from the environment for recognition.

Visual Object Recognition

Recognition of an object depends on the formation of a mental representation that is:

- three-dimensional
- independent of size, orientation, brightness or distance from the viewer
- sensitive to movement in different directions
- accessible to stored representations of the object in memory.

The access to stored representations of all the objects we have encountered can be compared to the recognition of a barcode at the supermarket checkout. However, this system would put an impossible overload on the storage of 'templates' in memory. The categorisation of items and storage of a central description of an object that represents a category, known as a prototype, lead to a more economical approach.

Top-down approaches in object recognition have emphasised the importance of contextual information. Textures, surfaces and lines in the visual environment give meaning to what we see, and these are interpreted in the context of the changing scene around us. Gibson (1979) proposed that surfaces and objects 'afford' action. The affordance of an object is what it offers as a possibility for action. A handle affords grasping, the shape of a jug affords tipping. Some people who have poor semantic knowledge of the meaning of objects can use them by activating the action system by a direct route from perception to action (Riddoch and Humphreys 1987). The importance of contextual information means that functional assessments in occupational therapy are facilitated in the patient's home environment using objects known to him or her. Performance is also affected by the number of objects present, the spatial arrangement of the objects, the complexity of the task and the environment (Toglia 1989).

Studies of object recognition have used laboratory experiments involving visual search and feature analysis, computer programs with algorithms which operate on two-dimensional images to reach a three-dimensional representation, and the assessment of patients with visual recognition problems to identify the stages in processing. The cognitive neuropsychology approach has produced an information processing model of object recognition (Ellis and Young 1988) which forms a useful basis for the assessment of object recognition problems in occupational therapy (Figure 6.5).

- Viewer-centred representation is the output of early visual perceptual processing. This representation is determined by the observer's viewpoint and this level is intact if the patient can copy line drawings and match objects.

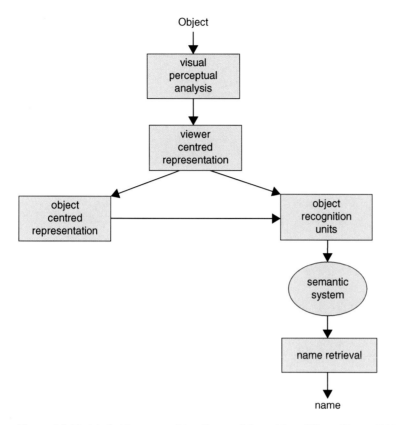

Figure 6.5 Model of object recognition. Source: Adapted from Ellis and Young (1988).

- Object-centred representation is the mental processing of objects which can be recognised in any view. This representation is independent of specific viewpoint. The level can be assessed by matching and recognition of the same object in different views.
- Object recognition units are stored descriptions of known objects in memory. The outputs from the viewer-centred and object-centred representations are compared with these stored descriptions for recognition of a known object.
- The semantic system is the processing of stored knowledge of the meaning and function of objects. The semantic representation may also be accessed from tactile input or from a verbal description of an object. If there is no deficit in the semantic system, objects can be matched by function, and can be used appropriately.
- Name retrieval is achieved by access to the lexicon of the names of known objects. Interruption at this level means that an object may be recognised and used, but cannot be named.

There is considerable evidence for the separation of structural, semantic and naming levels of processing in object recognition, with some cross-modular processing (known as cascade). Problems in the use of objects can arise due to impairment at any of these three levels.

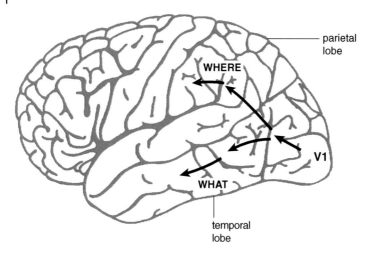

Figure 6.6 What and where pathways.

Naming problems require co-operation with a speech and language therapist. A person with a naming problem may be able to recognise objects by touch and he or she can mime their use. This is known as *optic aphasia*.

In Chapter 9, we will consider the output from semantics to the action system which activates the movements associated with the use of objects.

What and Where Pathways

Early visual perceptual processing occurs in the occipital lobe. In the 1980s, two independent projections were identified extending from the occipital lobe to the temporal and parietal lobes (Figure 6.6). Studies in neuropsychology have focused on the differences in processing in the two pathways.

- The ventral pathway extending to the temporal lobe relates to the perceptual processing of objects for recognition, known as the 'what' stream.
- The dorsal pathway to the posterior parietal lobe relates to the perceptual processing of the position of objects in space, known as the 'where' stream.

Case study (Goodale and Milner 1992)
DF aged 35 years had bilateral lesions in the occipital lobes as a result of the inhalation of carbon monoxide from a leaky gas heater. She was unable to recognise objects, drawings or pictures. She was able to name an object when it was put in her hands so it was not a naming problem. Also she had no loss of visual acuity. DF was assessed on her ability to perceive the orientation of a three-dimensional object. In this experiment, she was asked to view a circular wooden block with a slot cut in it. The orientation of the slot could be varied.

In the first condition, DF was given a card and asked to orient her hand so that the card fitted the slot, for example hold the card horizontal if the slot was horizontal. She was unable to do this, orienting her hand vertically for a horizontal slot. In the second condition DF was asked to insert the card into the slot. She was able to do this accurately, orienting her hand correctly before contact with the slot.

Goodale and Milner concluded that processing systems use two different sources of perceptual information, one to identify objects and the other to localise objects in space for guiding action. DF was able to respond to the visual processing that guided movement but was impaired in the route to the temporal lobe for object recognition. This case study provides evidence for the dissociation of object perception and object action.

More recent studies have shown that the guiding of action is limited to the uniaxial slot and does not apply when the action involves a shape with two axes. The difference between processing in the what and where pathways has been modified to include interaction between them and the inclusion of other modules. Some authors have also suggested that the dorsal pathway should be called the 'how' stream, describing its role in mediating action.

When the dorsal stream is impaired in patients with parietal lesions, they can recognise objects via the ventral stream but cannot use visual information to guide action for their use. This is known as *optic ataxia.* These patients have good object recognition but cannot use objects appropriately.

Visual Agnosia

Visual agnosia is the inability to recognise familiar objects by sight in the absence of any significant visual or intellectual impairment. Agnosia means literally 'no knowledge'. Pure agnosia is clinically rare but many single cases of visual object agnosia have been reported in cognitive neuropsychology.

Visual object agnosia was first divided into two main types by Lissauer in 1900.

- *Apperceptive agnosia* – a failure to form a stable perceptual representation of objects. Recognition problems are based on impairment of visual perception. Patients cannot match or copy shapes or objects. They are able to identify and name objects from touch and sound.
- *Associative* (semantic) *agnosia* – the inability to recognise familiar objects when visual perception is intact. Patients are able to copy and draw shapes and objects. They can name objects from verbal descriptions of their structure but cannot describe the function of objects. A mental representation can be formed but it cannot be associated with stored knowledge of objects and their use.

Apperceptive agnosia usually occurs in right hemisphere lesions and associative agnosia with left hemisphere lesions, particularly the left temporal lobe. Associative agnosia may be explained as a disruption of the 'what' pathway.

In the 1980s, more complex tests for visual agnosia were developed, for example presentation of objects in unusual views, with minimal features, in silhouette and superimposed shapes. Tests of object function have included matching a test item (rolled umbrella) with an object with the same function (open umbrella) or a visually similar object with a different function (walking stick). These studies have identified variations of the types of visual object agnosia within the two main divisions.

Case study (Humphreys and Riddoch 1987)

HJA had bilateral occipital lesions as a result of a stroke following an appendectomy. He could move around without bumping into objects and could reach out to pick things up but he was unable to recognise familiar objects from vision. He was able to identify objects by touch and to give detailed definitions of named objects. HJA could copy drawings, taking hours to draw them and producing considerable detail. His perception of the fine detail was intact but he was unable to relate them to the whole object for recognition. When he made an accurate copy of a line drawing of an owl, he said that he saw a complex pattern of lines and he could not identify the owl.

Based on comprehensive study of HJA, Humphreys and Riddoch proposed that in normal object recognition, the global form of an object is coded first and then the local fine detail is integrated into the form for recognition. Humpreys and Riddoch introduced the term *integrative agnosia.*

An account of object agnosia developed by Farah (1991) focused on whole- or part-based processing for recognition. Farah suggested that object recognition, which involves both whole- and part-based processing, lies in the middle of the continuum between face recognition (whole-based processing) and the recognition of words (part-based processing). This hypothesis is based on a review of all published cases in the literature. People with object agnosia often have either face agnosia or alexia in addition, but these other two conditions usually occur alone.

Some people with visual agnosia are able to recognise some objects better than others. Farah and other authors have reported individuals with agnosia who could name drawings of living things but could not name non-living items. These studies, supported by PET scan studies, have suggested that different processes or parts of the brain are involved in the recognition of living compared with non-living things. This observation is known as a category-specific impairment. So far, there has been no report of a double dissociation, i.e. a person who can recognise non-living but not living things. More recent research has pointed to the use of line drawings for stimuli in these tests as the source of the apparent category specificity. Living things are items that are more familiar as words than images, and drawings of them are more complex than those of non-living things.

It is difficult to imagine the problems confronting people with agnosia who are surrounded by a very confused visual environment. For some, nothing seems familiar and basic forms blend into confusion. For others, the detail of objects obscures the outline form. This may be like looking through a telescope and trying to remember the view in different directions. Some people show a marked recovery in the first few months after onset. For others, the problem persists for the rest of their lives. Interesting accounts can be read in Humphreys and Riddoch (1987) and Sacks (1985).

The relationship between visual perceptual deficits and the performance of activities of daily living (ADL) in stroke patients has been investigated (Edmans and Lincoln 1990; Titus *et al.* 1991; Toglia 1989). The nature and number of perceptual tests used in each of the studies are different but the results predict that the presence of visual perceptual deficits in right or left hemisphere lesion patients does affect ADL performance adversely. The ability of tests of visual perception to predict outcome, either at admission or discharge, is less clear, however. Donnelly (2002) found no relationship between scores on the RPAB and functional performance at admission to hospital for stroke patients, but the presence or absence of visual perceptual deficit, combined with age, were the two factors found to significantly predict functional performance at discharge (greater age was negatively correlated with scores on the Adult Functional Independence Measure).

Face Recognition

The ability to recognise faces has great significance in the way we function in everyday living. Face recognition is the basis of all our interaction with other people. A face offers much more information than an object. In common with objects, a face must be processed as a visual structure and recognised as a face when seen from different views. The detail of the size, shape of the eyes, nose and mouth, and the texture of the skin make each face unique and familiar. In a face, we are also presented with the expression of feelings and emotion, and with the movement of the lips in speech. Very early in development, a young baby makes movements of the eyes and head to follow the face of someone in his or her view and may copy their facial expressions. We can identify a family member, a friend or a colleague from the sound of his or her voice, from a fleeting glimpse in a crowd or from their unique facial expressions. The recognition of a person is supported by the integration of knowledge about the person, for example age, gender, occupation and behaviour. There are many different reasons for a failure to recognise someone but we always need to know who they are before we can remember their name.

Studies in neuropsychology have focused on the question: 'Is face recognition special and different from objects?'. Some support for the distinct processing for faces is offered by studies using face inversion.

Activity

Ask a partner to lie supine on the floor and then look at the face from a position behind his or her head. Try the same situation with objects lying on a table, viewing each in normal and inverted position from the top end of the table. What difference do you notice in the view of the upside-down face compared with a reversed object?

When photographs of famous people are presented to normal subjects in normal and inverted orientation, recognition is instant for the upright position but slower when inverted. This inversion effect is much less marked with objects. The results of imaging

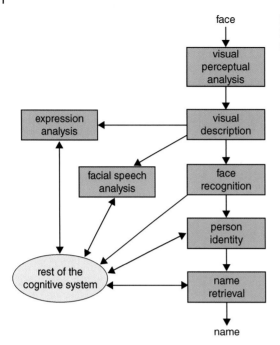

face

Figure 6.7 Model of face recognition. Source: Adapted from Bruce and Young (1986).

studies on normal people have shown that different areas of the temporal lobe are activated when upright faces are recognised compared with inverted ones. These observations suggest that templates in memory are stored separately for upright and inverted faces.

Early studies of the stages of processing in cognitive neuropsychology, based on studies of normal people and those with problems in recognising familiar faces, led to a model of face recognition described by Bruce and Young (1986). More recent investigations have focused on the detail of the parallel processing of biographical information. The model shown in Figure 6.7 is based on the Bruce and Young model.

The stages of processing are as follows.

- Visual perceptual analysis discriminates the visual elements of a face: the eyes, the nose, the mouth and so on. Disruption at this early stage means inability to distinguish the basic features of a face, and is likely to lead to more widespread perceptual difficulties.
- Visual structural description discriminates a face as different from objects and other items shown by the ability to match faces. Parallel processing in modules for expression analysis and facial speech movements (lip reading) occurs at this level.
- Face recognition units contain structural information about known faces. This allows for the identification of a known face but not a particular person. *Is this a face that looks familiar?*
- The person identity nodes are stored knowledge of the identity of particular known people. *Do I know this person?* The output from the processing of facial expressions and facial speech, together with biographical information of age, culture, occupation and so on, accesses this level via the semantic system and memory (labelled the cognitive system).

- Name retrieval is the stage of access to stored knowledge of the names of known people. *I know this person, what is his or her name?* Disruption at this stage means the person has been identified but cannot be named.

The model shows that name generation can only be accessed from the person identity nodes which in turn store biographical information about the person. This means that we are not able to put a name to a face without knowing other information about that person, for example occupation or relationships. This was confirmed by a study which asked people to keep a diary of problems they experienced in face recognition (Young *et al.* 1985). The subjects never reported putting a name to a face while at the same time knowing nothing else about the person. Only a few subjects could remember some information about a person but not their name.

Activity

Over a short lunchtime break in the refectory at college or work, look carefully at everyone around you. Keep a total count and note (a) how many you can recognise, (b) how many you can name and (c) how many are unfamiliar.

What factors determine your ability to recognise or name the members of this group?

Prosopagnosia

Prosopagnosia is the inability to recognise familiar faces in the absence of sensory impairment. In severe cases, the person cannot recognise their own family or even their own reflection. A face may be recognised as a face but not whose face it is. Sometimes, family members are not forgotten and they are recognised when the voice is heard. Loss of naming must be differentiated from pure memory loss so co-operation with the speech and language therapist is important.

The parallel processing of facial expressions and facial speech occurs independently from recognition based on the visual structural representation. This dissociation has been shown in people who were able to recognise the expressions of faces they could not recognise while others showed the opposite. They could not identify the expression on a face they could recognise. We need to be able to recognise a face whatever the expression at the time. There is a similar dissociation between expression analysis and lip reading.

Another interesting line of research into face recognition is the phenomenon of covert recognition. People who are totally unable to recognise faces have demonstrated that some recognition is occurring below the level of conscious awareness. When prosopagnosic subjects were asked to learn to associate names with faces, they found it much easier to learn to associate a face with its real name than with some other name, demonstrating some unconscious recognition.

Face recognition is based on a modular system of independent processes which can be selectively impaired. PET scan studies have identified the right temporal lobe when specific faces were identified by normal subjects. Single case studies of people with prosopagnosia in the literature showed bilateral damage in the occipital and temporal lobes or unilateral damage in the same lobes on the right side.

Stereognosis: Tactile Gnosis

Much has been researched and written about visual spatial perception and visual agnosias, but agnosia in other sensory modalities also occurs and can create significant difficulties for people, affecting their functional independence, safety and performance in a wide range of occupations. Because so much research and clinical attention is directed to impairments of the visual perceptual system, agnosias in other modalities risk being ignored or their impact on function and quality of life underestimated. When brain injury results in primary somatosensory deficits, the potential for tactile perceptual deficits may be overlooked. When motor impairments are present, the focus in rehabilitation may be on recovery of motor function without recognition of the possibility of primary sensory deficits or tactile agnosia contributing to poor performance and lack of progress in recovery.

Stereognosis (also termed tactile gnosis or haptic recognition) is the process of perception and recognition of objects and their properties by touch alone. This requires the sensory processing of information about an object – texture, firmness, size, spatial aspects and temperature – to form a tactile representation which can then be compared to stored semantic knowledge about the object, to enable recognition. We depend upon tactile gnosis to identify objects that we cannot see (e.g. searching for keys in a bag or locating a light switch in the dark), for navigating and interacting with our immediate environment when it is out of visual field or we cannot direct our vision to it (e.g. sitting down in a chair, operating the controls of a car) and for manipulating and orientating objects appropriately for use (e.g. holding a pen to write, tying a necktie).

Tactile gnosis requires processing and integration of cutaneous and proprioceptive sensations. The latter provides information on the shape and position of the hands and the movements the joints and muscles are producing in manipulating the object, contributing knowledge of surface resilience, spatial properties and moving parts. Manipulation of objects in hand is therefore an important ability, requiring dexterity, and it follows that difficulties with praxis (see Chapter 9) may contribute to poor tactile gnosis.

Tactile Agnosia: Astereognosis

As with visual gnosis, tactile gnosis involves a number of stages: basic sensory processing, sensory integration and semantic association. An agnosia may occur due to disruption of integration, termed *apperceptive* tactile agnosia, or due to disruption of acquisition of meaning, termed *associative* tactile agnosia.

Case studies of individuals with unilateral cerebral hemisphere damage have demonstrated that tactile agnosia most often arises from damage to the parietal and occipito-temporal cortices. It rarely occurs in isolation from other cognitive perceptual difficulties, and there are very few assessments specific to it and very limited data concerning its treatment.

Functional Consequences of Agnosias

For people with visual perceptual deficits, the world is seen as unfamiliar, strange and confusing. In the home environment, activities of daily living are difficult to perform when objects cannot be recognised. The appropriate tool cannot be selected for a particular purpose. Food containers in cupboards cannot be selected by shape and colour. In dressing, items of clothing cannot be chosen particularly when they are overlapping and lying on a bed cover. Clothes may not be recognised when they are upside down or inside out. There may be difficulty in recognising personal possessions, such as the contents of a handbag. The enjoyment of walking around the abundance of flowers in the garden is less than before.

In the outside world, items cannot be identified on the supermarket shelves and there may be difficulty in sorting coins for payment at the checkout. In the street, the speed and distance of moving vehicles cannot be estimated accurately enough for safety. The pursuit of leisure activities may be marred by inability to estimate the distance of the flight of a ball.

Poor face recognition affects social interaction with family, friends and neighbours and leads to social isolation. Advice to relatives and friends on the importance of the voice and facial expressions can reduce the stress for the person.

Agnosias in the tactile, auditory and olfactory modalities also affect daily living. Tactile agnosia leads to difficulties when activities have to be done out of view. Doing up a back fastener on clothes or finding coins in a pocket are examples of this. Work activities using equipment and machines often involve manipulative operations out of view. Auditory agnosia can lead to inability to distinguish the voices of different people. The person may leave the vacuum cleaner or the TV on, and complain that the hearing aid is broken. Olfactory agnosia has implications for safety when the smell of gas, smoke or burnt food is ignored.

Suggestions for Assessment and Intervention

Assessment

- Basic sensory abilities (visual, somatosensory) and basic perceptual processing must be assessed prior to more complex cognitive functions. In particular, it is important to be able to differentiate problems of perceptual processing from primary sensory deficits. Loss of visual field or acuity can significantly affect function. Object agnosia may manifest as inappropriate use of objects in a task, also seen in apraxia. Sensory loss in the hand may mask a tactile agnosia.
- Use the normal environment to screen for basic visual perceptual deficits; for example, ask the person to select all the mugs of the same colour or size from a cupboard (visual scanning, colour and shape matching); to select one specific item from pile of clothes and identify buttons and pockets on it (figure ground).
- For tactile agnosia, having first screened for cutaneous and proprioceptive loss, the main assessment method (non-standardised) is to present a series of objects familiar

to the person, with vision occluded, and ask him to identify them by touch alone, picking up and manipulating them in hand. This should be done with each hand in turn. Objects such as keys, comb, pen, paper clip, ball can be used. Accuracy is scored by counting the number of correct identifications divided by the total number of objects. A 'normal' response would be full accuracy with each object identified within a few seconds.

- Observe the person whilst undertaking daily activities in the normal environment, for the functional impact of impairments in tasks such as:
  - recognising friends and relatives by sight (prosopagnosia)
  - locating named objects in a room (object recognition and naming)
  - finding several of the same item placed in different orientations (object constancy)
  - undertaking tasks using several objects (object agnosia)
  - locating items in a handbag without looking.
- Record the type and frequency of errors in task performance, at what point a task breaks down and the context.
- Use components of standardised assessments to detect and measure specific visual perceptual deficits, and any change over time.

Assessment Resources

A range of standardised assessments of perceptual function exist and are appropriate for use by occupational therapists. The RPAB, COTNAB and LOTCA (see assessment list at the end of Chapter 2) contain tests of visual perception, sometimes in combination with tests of motor or other cognitive abilities. Cooke *et al.* (2005) developed the Occupational Therapy Adult Perceptual Screening Test (OT-APST) for visual perception in adult stroke and brain injury. Quintana's chapter on assessing vision, visual perception and praxis in Radomski and Trombly Latham (2008) addresses the assessment of visual foundation skills such as visual field and oculomotor control, and basic visual perception.

Stereognosis receives relatively little attention in assessment or intervention. Gillen (2011) briefly mentions intervention but not assessment. Bentzel's chapter on assessment of sensation in Radomski and Trombly Latham (2008) includes stereognosis.

In general, limited attention seems to be given to separating sensory from perceptual components in tactile object recognition, but can be important for properly understanding an individual's functional difficulties. Differentiating basic sensory status from tactile recognition and semantic knowledge of objects will enable identification of any perceptual deficit and, subsequently, correctly focused interventions.

Intervention

- Methods of remediation may include repeated blocked practice of exercises such as locating and naming objects, colour and shape matching, and scanning across the visual field for objects in a variety of places. Computer programs and worksheets can be used for figure ground and scanning exercises.
- There is limited evidence to support the value of programmes of remediation, in terms of the extent to which such practice carries over into functional improvement. Practice regimes may result in improvement only in highly similar tasks (near transfer) and not generalise to daily life. Grading occurs by increasing the number or variety of objects, the complexity and variety of contexts, and the reduction of cues given during tasks.

- The naming, locating and identifying of objects and people can be incorporated into daily routines, both to maximise remediation and to assist adaptation by the association of objects and people with environments.
- Tactile agnosia can be compensated for by the use of other sensory modalities – visual, olfactory or auditory – to recognise objects. To support improvement of stereognosis, the person might start practising identifying simple shapes by touch, combining tactile with visual recognition (Gillen 2011).
- Adaptation to the environment and task objects, and use of compensatory techniques are important to optimise independent and safe function.
  - Providing objects and tools in specific colours to enable object recognition by association with colour (e.g. all mugs in bright yellow).
  - Identifying objects by touch (intact stereognosis).
  - Encouraging others to identify themselves verbally at each meeting.
  - Ensuring the normal environment is uncluttered and organised consistently so that objects can be located easily.
- Family involvement is very important. Participation and co-operation with adaptive measures carried over into the home can increase the individual's independence. Understanding the nature of the visual perceptual deficits will enable family members to continue to devise and refine strategies for existing and novel situations in the future.

Sources of evidence

Quintana and Bentzel, in Radomski and Trombly Latham (2008), describe interventions for visual, visual perceptual and sensory impairments respectively following neurological damage. Gillen (2011) considers approaches to and techniques for intervention for cognitive and perceptual impairments following stroke. Lee *et al.* (2001) mention the need to incorporate both remedial and adaptive approaches and techniques to optimise functional independence.

SUMMARY

1) Visual acuity, the area of the visual field and the control of eye movements are known as the basic visual functions. The ability to scan the features of the space around us demands an adequate area of intact visual fields, pursuit and saccadic movements of the eyes and shifts of attention.
2) Early visual processing includes colour, depth, figure ground and motion. There is evidence for separable perceptual processing of shape and motion. Perceptual constancy allows shapes and objects viewed in a variety of conditions to be perceived as the same.
3) Theories of visual perception have been developed to identify processing from the analysis of the retinal image to recognition. Other top-down processing theories emphasise the importance of past experience. Sensory input is processed in terms of our expectations about the visual world.
4) The visual processing of objects follows two parallel processing streams from the occipital lobe. The 'what' stream, extending to the posterior parietal lobe, operates on early visual processing for object recognition and accesses stored memories of related objects. The 'where' stream, extending to the temporal lobe, processes spatial information related to objects and mediates the guiding of action related to objects.

5) Modular models of object recognition show three main stages of processing in series: structural description; semantic representation of the meaning and function of objects; and naming. Each of these levels can be selectively impaired.

6) Accounts of visual object agnosia have described two main types: apperceptive agnosia, a failure to form a stable perceptual representation of objects; and associative agnosia, the inability to integrate the perceptual representation of objects with their function. More recent accounts of object agnosia emphasise the separation of global or whole-based processing from that related to the detail of the parts.

7) A model of face recognition describes a modular system with stages from visual structural encoding to person identity and naming, with additional parallel modules for facial expression and facial speech processed via the semantic system. Person identity also includes knowledge of biographical information, for example age, gender, culture and occupation.

8) Perceptual processing occurs in other sensory modalities, enabling us to make sense of gustatory, olfactory, auditory and somatic sensory information. Agnosia can occur in all of these modalities. Tactile agnosia, or astereognosis, rarely occurs in isolation and can be masked by or mistaken for primary sensory deficit. It has significant functional consequences in daily life, and must be screened for and identified if interventions are to be appropriately focused.

References

Andrewes, D. (2001) *Disorders of perception, in Neuropsychology: From Theory to Practice*, Psychology Press, Hove.

Bruce, V. and Young, A.W. (1986) Understanding face recognition. *Journal of Psychology*, **77**, 305–327.

Cate, Y. and Richards, L. (2000) Relationship between performance on tests of basic visual functions and visual-perceptual processing in persons after brain injury. *American Journal of Occupational Therapy*, **54** (3), 326–334.

Cooke, D.M., McKenna, K. and Fleming, J. (2005) Development of a standardized occupational therapy screening tool for visual perception in adults. *Scandinavian Journal of Occupational Therapy*, **12** (2), 59–71.

Donnelly, S. (2002) The Rivermead Perceptual Assessment Battery: can it predict functional performance? *Australian Occupational Therapy Journal*, **49**, 71–81.

Edmans, J.A. and Lincoln, N.B. (1990) The relationship between perceptual deficits after stroke and independence in activities of daily living. *British Journal of Occupational Therapy*, **53**, 139–142.

Ellis, A.W. and Young, A.W. (1988) *Human Cognitive Neuropsychology*, Lawrence Erlbaum, London.

Farah, M.J. (1991) Patterns of co-occurrence among associative agnosias: implications for visual object representation. *Cognitive Neuropsychology*, **8**, 1–19.

Gibson, J.J. (1979) *The Ecological Approach to Visual Perception*, Houghton Mifflin, Boston, Massachusetts.

Gillen, G. (2011) *Stroke Rehabilitation: A Function-based Approach*, 3rd edn, Mosby, St Louis, Missouri.

Goodale, M.A. and Milner, A.D. (1992) Separate visual pathways for perception and action. *Trends in Neurosciences*, **15**, 20–25.

Humphreys, G.W. and Riddoch, M.J. (1987) *To See or Not to See. A Case Study of visual Agnosia*, Lawrence Erlbaum, London.

Lee, S.S., Powell, N. and Esdaile, S. (2001) A functional model of cognitive rehabilitation in occupational therapy. *Canadian Journal of Occupational Therapy*, **68** (1), 41–50.

Lotery, A.J., Wiggam, M.I., Jackson, A.J. et al. (2000) Correctable visual impairment in stroke rehabilitation patients. *Age and Ageing*, **29**, 221–222.

Radomski, M.V. and Trombly Latham, C.A. (eds) (2008) *Occupational Therapy for Physical Dysfunction*, 6th edn, Lippincott, Williams and Wilkins, Philadelphia.

Riddoch, M.J. and Humphreys, G.W. (1987) Visual object processing in a case of optic aphasia: a case of semantic access agnosia. *Cognitive Neuropsychology*, **4**, 131–185.

Sacks, O. (1985) *The Man Who Mistook His Wife for a Hat*, Duckworth, London.

Sand, K.M., Midelfart, A., Thomassen, L., Melms, A., Wilhelm, H. and Hoff, J.M. (2013) Visual impairment in stroke patients – a review. *Acta Neurologica Scandinavica*, **127** (Suppl. 196), 52–56.

Titus, M.N.D., Gall, N.G., Yerxa, E.J., Roberson, T.A. and Mack, W. (1991) Correlation of perceptual performance and activities of daily living in stroke patients. *American Journal of Occupational Therapy*, **45**, 410–418.

Toglia, J.P. (1989) Visual perception of objects. An approach to assessment and intervention. *American Journal of Occupational Therapy*, **43**, 587–595.

Young, A.W., Hay, D.C. and Ellis, A.W. (1985) The faces that launched a thousand slips: everyday difficulties and errors in recognizing people. *British Journal of Psychology*, **76**, 495–523.

Zihl, J., von Cramen, D. and Mai, N. (1983) Selective disturbance of movement vision after bilateral brain damage. *Brain*, **106**, 313–340.

7

Complex Perceptual Functions: Body Scheme and Agnosia, Constructional Skills and Neglect

Stephanie Tempest and Linda Maskill

AIMS

1) To consider the concept of body scheme, in contrast to body image. To define some of the body scheme disorders, including the agnosias, and their functional implications.
2) To explore the demands placed upon our spatial perceptual system by constructional activities and the difficulties caused by constructional deficits.
3) To critically debate the nature of neglect, its functional impact and the lived experience of the impairment.
4) To outline some suggestions for assessment and intervention.

In Chapter 6, we were introduced to the building blocks and components which enable sensory processing. This chapter will consider some of the complex functions which arise from the basic perceptual processes as well as the functional manifestations and consequences following damage to the brain.

Spatial ability is 'knowing where things are'. As we move around, we scan the area of space offered by the visual field of both our eyes. Once a surface or an object has been located, we analyse its relation both to our own body and to other objects around. We may draw upon other sensory skills to enable further analysis, for example feel a drinking cup to distinguish if it is made of glass or plastic. In the use of objects in functional activities, these spatial relations are integrated with the movements of the arm in reaching space. Constructional activities, i.e. units assembled into a two- or three-dimensional whole, have a large spatial component. We may be unaware of our own spatial abilities until we try to assemble a new kitchen gadget or an item of flat-packed furniture.

On a larger scale, the position of buildings and landmarks is important in finding our way around on foot, on a bicycle or in a car. The spatial relations of the features of the environment are integrated with whole-body movement. We need to discriminate right and left, and be able to mentally rotate a pathway to follow it in different directions.

Neuropsychology for Occupational Therapists: Cognition in Occupational Performance, Fourth Edition.
Edited by Linda Maskill and Stephanie Tempest.
© 2017 John Wiley & Sons Ltd. Published 2017 by John Wiley & Sons Ltd.
Companion Website: www.wiley.com/go/maskill/neuropsychologyOT

Yet, spatial processing in everyday living has not been investigated to the same extent as other elements of perception. One reason may be the complex nature of spatial perception and difficulty in separating the spatial element from other cognitive abilities. Attention and memory are also involved in the exploration of different areas of space. There is some evidence of separable systems for visual and spatial perception with interaction between them; some of this evidence will be revisited in Chapter 9 when considering purposeful movement and apraxia. The specific loss of the ability to locate seen objects is rare and it is usually accompanied by visual perceptual problems. The spatial component becomes obvious in tasks that require assembling parts together to construct a whole.

Spatial abilities demand an adequate visual field and the control of eye movements. The basic visual functions were described in detail in Chapter 6. This chapter will begin by considering complex perception at the body level, including body scheme and some of the agnosias, and then we will critically consider the role of spatial skills in our constructional abilities. The chapter will end with a detailed exploration of neglect from a sensory and premotor perspective. Suggestions for assessment and intervention will draw this chapter to a close.

Body Scheme

The body scheme is the knowledge of the position of the parts of the body and the spatial relationship between them; it is constantly updated through movement. This knowledge is based on the integration of perceptual processing of the input from vision, proprioception, tactile and pressure sensation, in all the parts of the body, as we move around. The discrimination of the direction of movements into upward and downward movements, right and left and so on is part of the body scheme.

The concept of the body scheme has not been well defined in the literature and no unified theoretical framework for it has been developed. Theories which describe the construction of the body scheme have supported either a mental representation that is innate or one that is developed from sensory feedback. It is not necessarily a conscious way in which we view ourselves.

In contrast, body image is a conscious representation of us; it relies on emotional and environmental inputs which produce a representation of our own body in visual imagery. This representation is often not the same as the exact physical appearance of our own body. When normal subjects are asked to draw a picture of themselves, the relative sizes of some body features may be larger or smaller than they really are. A disorder of body image has additional psychosocial and emotional factors.

There are several different mental representations which are incorporated into the processing of body knowledge (Sirigu 1991), including the following.

- The lexical (name) and semantic (function) representation of each body part. *The hand is used for grasping.*
- The structural description of the position of each part in the body. *The hand is at the end of the arm.*
- The spatiotemporal representation of the changing positions of body parts. *The hand is moving across the body.*

Disorders of Body Scheme

Body scheme disorder is not a single deficit and may present in different forms. The functional loss may be bilateral or only one side of the body may be affected. Damage to the parietal lobe, the site of somatosensory integration and the termination of the 'where' pathway, has been implicated in body scheme disorder.

The classification of disorders of body scheme is problematic and there is some disagreement about which disorders relate purely to the body scheme without the inclusion of other perceptual deficits. Descriptions in the literature relate to the symptoms presented rather than the specific cognitive processing that is disrupted.

Agnosia

This section describes some of the 'agnosias', i.e. the inability to interpret specific sensory information, causing objects, smells or sounds to essentially be devoid of meaning.

- *Somatognosia* is a failure to recognise the parts of the body and to perceive their relative positions in space. The person with somatognosia has poor balance and equilibrium. Movements are inaccurate in the presence of normal proprioception.
- *Right/left discrimination deficit* is the inability to distinguish right and left in the symmetrical parts of the body. Confusion of right and left may be part of somatognosia. Many normal subjects have difficulty in right/left discrimination, particularly when asked to point to parts of body shapes presented in unconventional orientations.
- Anosognosia is the denial of the severity or even the presence of an affected limb. When asked to move the limb, the commands are often ignored, and various reasons are offered as an excuse. One subject called his arm George after his son who didn't work! The person is in danger of injury to the limb. Anosognosia may be part of severe unilateral neglect or body scheme disorder.
- Autopagnosia is an inability to identify the parts of the body. Finger agnosia is when this is only related to the fingers. Autopagnosia may be a naming problem associated with aphasia.

Disorders of body scheme affect all personal care activities. Difficulty in manipulating objects in contact with the body presents difficulties in washing, toileting and dressing. Clothes may be worn inside out or back to front. Only one half of the body may be dressed. In anosognosia, there is a danger of harming the body part that is ignored. People with right/left discrimination deficit have problems with using equipment that is direction oriented. In locomotion, the negotiation of stairs and kerbs is difficult without the knowledge of the distance moved by the lower limbs at each step. This particularly affects visually impaired people since they have to rely heavily on body scheme and proprioception to estimate the depth of stairs.

The agnosias extend beyond the body as some people present with visuospatial agnosia, which distorts the perception of the physical and social dimensions of both the person's own body and the environment. At the person level, kerbs and stairs present a hazard for tripping and falling. Utensils are dropped off the edge of work surfaces or tables. In dressing, there may be difficulty in distinguishing the top, bottom, inside and outside of clothing.

A person in a wheelchair will have problems in transferring when he or she cannot judge the distance between wheelchair and the toilet or bed. Wheelchair training is very difficult when the person cannot estimate distances, or turn to the right or left appropriately. The person who is ambulant may not find the way from one location to another.

Constructional Skills

In constructional activities, single units are organised into a two- or three-dimensional whole. The construction may be simply putting our clothes on in the morning. Preparing a meal has a constructional component when making a sandwich or laying the table. More complex constructional skill is needed to assemble a doll's house or flat-packed furniture. There are many constructional elements in maintenance and repair tasks, such as fixing a bicycle or a lawn mower.

During the assembly of units to make a whole, the location of items in the environment must be integrated with the extent and direction of hand movements. The mental operations of spatial location engage the dorsal 'where' pathway ending in the parietal lobe described in Chapter 6. This spatial information accesses the motor areas of the frontal lobe for planning and execution of the movements. In the evaluation of constructional ability, the main difficulty is in isolating the spatial component from the motor component of the task. A further problem occurs for people with left hemisphere lesions (right hemiplegia) when the non-dominant hand may have to be used. The instructions for assembly in construction tasks need to be visual for the person with right hemiplegia and verbal in left hemiplegia.

The investigation of constructional skills has centred around the analysis of two types of activity: drawing and building/assembly. In drawing tasks, the person is asked to copy elaborate line drawings from a model or to draw from memory. In two- or three-dimensional tasks, subjects are asked to assemble coloured wooden blocks into specific designs, or build a three-dimensional construction from component blocks of different shapes and sizes, for example the constructional task in the standardised Rivermead Perceptual Assessment Battery. The results are examined for clearly defined errors.

Errors made in two-dimensional line drawings by right compared with left brain-damaged people are as follows.

- People with right brain damage produce drawings that are disorganised with distortion of the spatial relationships. Fragmented outlines are drawn with extra or repeated strokes.
- People with left brain damage simplify the drawings and leave elements out. Sometimes the overall spatial layout is preserved but the drawing is lacking in detail.

Deficits in constructional ability affect all instrumental activities of daily living at some level. Meal preparation, shopping and house cleaning present problems particularly when electrical or mechanical equipment is used. Household gadgets reduce muscular effort and joint strain but the cognitive components of the task increase when the labour-saving devices have to be assembled. Dressing is a constructional task that involves holding the garments in the correct orientation to the body. Gardening has a major spatial component for handling seeds and planting an array of bedding plants. The use of cash machines demands knowledge of the layout of the key pad and the position of the slot for inserting the card. Using a smartphone requires the ability to use the touchscreen to activate a specific app. Many leisure pursuits, including all ball games, require the ability to track moving targets and locate the position of other members of a team.

Neglect

Neglect is another disorder related to impairment of spatial abilities. The person with neglect fails to report, respond or orient to stimuli in the space contralateral to the side of the brain damage, usually the left. The majority of cases of neglect are seen in people with right parietal lobe damage, which leads to neglect of the left side of space, but right side neglect has been reported.

People with neglect live and act in only one half of their surroundings. In the early stages, they may have little insight into their problems and report the world as if it were complete. For some, the left half of the body feels incomplete. Spontaneous non-use movements of the left hand may occur but no functional movements are made. In dressing with T-shirt and trousers, only the right arm and right leg are dressed. Men with neglect shave only one side of the face. Food preparation is difficult and only food on the right side of the plate is eaten. Reading a book is difficult when the words on the left side of the page are ignored. It may be easier to follow the information from items in a newspaper which are presented in columns on the page.

An ambulant person or wheelchair user may always follow a route turning to the right, and bump into things on the left. Problems occur in social interaction when any person approaching or sitting on the left is ignored. The box below details the lived experience of neglect.

The lived experience of neglect (adapted from Tham *et al.* 2000)

My body feels new and unfamiliar. If I touch my left shoulder, I can remind myself that my arm and hand actually belong to me and are not just objects, like five sausages just sitting there for a hand.

It is also so difficult when, one minute, I'm having dinner with my husband and the next he has disappeared from my view. I feel like such a failure when I hear another crash and then realise the wheelchair has gone into the wall again.

But then, over time, I gradually start to feel that I must take responsibility for this arm, like I'm carrying a baby that I can never put down. And I start to search for an anchor on the left side so I know where I am; but sometimes, I just need a bit of time to do this. I now tell myself 'look to the left, look to the left' – it's engraved in my brain.

There is much debate and little consensus on the definition of types of neglect. Current thinking views it as a spatial, rather than attentional, difficulty. Some researchers distinguish between sensory neglect (a challenge at the input stage of perceptual processing) and premotor neglect (towards the output stage of gesture production). In the latter, the person fails to orientate their limbs to the contralesional hemispace (for further detail on the current concepts of neglect see Ting *et al.* 2011).

With regard to sensory neglect, this may occur in the tactile, auditory, olfactory or visual modalities. Furthermore, visual neglect can be divided into different spatial domains: personal, peripersonal or extrapersonal space (Figure 7.1). There are case study descriptions of people who present with impaired personal neglect only, warranting a debate that there are different underlying anatomies; for example, some researchers suggest the major mechanism for personal neglect is deficient body representation (Baas *et al.* 2011). A disorder of body representation thus places the impairment within the domain of spatial perception rather than a deficit of attention.

To appreciate the perceptual nature of neglect is to understand the concept of relative salience. A person with neglect may not be able to locate an object on the left if is small or insignificant in comparison to the other objects in the locality. However, a larger framed photograph of a loved one, thus attaching emotion and meaning, may be located on the left if surrounded by smaller objects of no personal relevance. There are implications for assessment here whereby people on a busy, acute hospital ward may not perform at their best if asked to locate an object on an already cluttered left-hand side (Gorgoraptis and Husain 2011).

Studies in neuropsychology have been largely concerned with visual neglect. Visual neglect must not be confused with a primary visual sensory deficit. The diagnosis of neglect can only be made after screening for sensory, visual field and primary motor deficits. Some people with visual neglect also have a visual field defect, for example a hemianopia which is compensated by moving the head, but others do not. In some cases, the neglect resolves after a few weeks but the persistence of severe neglect is a poor prognostic indicator, for people with right brain damage, in terms of their ability to respond to rehabilitation.

Extinction is a phenomenon commonly found in neglect. This can be demonstrated by asking the person to close their eyes and then touch both their hands simultaneously. Touch is then only reported on one side. When either hand is touched in isolation, the person does report it. Extinction can occur in response to visual, auditory or tactile

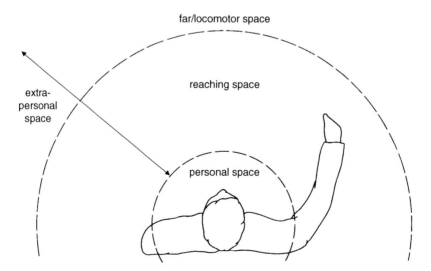

Figure 7.1 Fractionation of space into personal, peripersonal and locomotor space.

stimuli, thus confirming the multisensory nature of neglect, even though the research focus remains on arguably the most tangible aspect which is visual neglect.

Neglect as a Disorder of Perception

Our perception of the world around us depends on the formation and storage of spatial representations of external space. Also, with our eyes closed, we can imagine a known external space; for example, we can explore a scene we experienced on holiday. Athletes in training can use visual imagery to mentally rehearse their performance in a particular event, for example to start sprinting on the 'b' of the 'bang' from the starter's pistol. The formation of mental representations occurs after basic perceptual analysis and before the execution of action in that space. It has been proposed that people with neglect are unable to form the mental representation of one side of space, although not all of them show imaginal neglect as well.

In a classic study of people with neglect, Bisiach and Luzatti (1978) presented the theory that people with right hemisphere damage are unable to activate the visual and spatial representations of items present in the contralateral hemispace. This means they may not be able to describe or think about that side of space.

In a case study (Bisiach and Luzatti 1978), two people with left side neglect were asked to imagine that they were in the Piazza del Duomo in Milan, which was well known to them. When they imagined standing in the square at the end facing the cathedral, they described in detail all the buildings on the right side of the square, but the buildings on the left were omitted. Next, they imagined they were standing at the opposite end of the square on the steps of the cathedral. Now they described all the buildings that they had neglected before, and omitted the buildings that were now on the left side. In each case, Bisiach and Luzatti explained this as an inability to activate the mental representations of the buildings on the left side of space and the consequent loss of visual imagery for the features on that side.

Similar accounts have been described more recently by clinicians studying people with neglect. For example, a lorry driver was asked to imagine he was driving up and down the M1 motorway. When driving north, he described all the landmarks on the right side of the motorway and omitted those on the left. When driving south, he recalled all the landmarks he had previously omitted and neglected those which now appeared on the left.

These examples support the theory that in right hemisphere damage, the mental representations of the left external space cannot be activated, thus causing the features of neglect.

The Role of Premotor Programming in Neglect (Premotor Neglect)

So far, we have focused on the sensory and spatial aspects of neglect. However, at the start of this section, we also considered the concept of premotor neglect which now warrants further exploration. In premotor neglect, movements are not made to the contralateral side even though there may be some awareness of a stimulus (Ting *et al.* 2011). This raises the possibility that neglect originates in the loss of processing in the premotor areas which initiate movement towards the affected side. This impairment is also sometimes referred to as hypokinesia.

Support for this theory comes from the demonstration that active movements of the limbs on the left side of the body in left hemispace can have an effect on the manifestation of neglect (Maddicks *et al.* 2003; Robertson and North 1992; Robertson *et al.* 1998). This is the theoretical basis from which limb activation therapy derives, i.e. a prediction that left limb movements activate the premotor area of the damaged right hemisphere which facilitates the initiation of movement to the left hemispace.

Limb activation therapy studies have used pencil and paper tests and more functional activities for the assessment of neglect. The effects of treatment have shown short-term reduction in neglect but the long-term generalisation to functional skills in daily living has not been demonstrated. Indeed, there remains a paucity of studies, compounded by a lack of research funding, which focus on effective rehabilitation strategies for neglect (Kerkhoff and Schenk 2012).

Therefore, there is currently no single theoretical account of neglect or a gold standard from which to assess and intervene. In standard assessments of neglect, it is difficult to separate perceptual and premotor aspects of the condition. The representational theory links sensory neglect to loss of high-level spatial processing. Premotor neglect is based on a deficit in the premotor system for the initiation of movement to the affected hemispace. However, in addition, both spatial processing and the initiation of movement rely on the recruitment of attention to that space.

Suggestions for Assessment and Intervention

Assessment

- Observe the individual in a variety of tasks and activities appropriate to his functional level, and record the type and frequency of errors made.
- For body scheme and/or neglect disorders, ask the person to point to body parts or touch one body part with another. In functional activities, observe for signs that the person is ignoring body parts such as when washing and dressing.
- Tasks used to assess constructional ability include laying the table, preparing a sandwich and assembling equipment such as a food processor or vacuum cleaner.
- Many visual spatial tasks are complex and demand memory, attention and problem-solving skills (executive functions). These may need to be assessed.
- Standardised assessments include measures of spatial and constructional abilities, body scheme and neglect.
- Pencil and paper tests for neglect include cancellation tasks. The person is asked to cross out a specific target shape, for example a large star, repeated over both sides of a page amongst distractors of different sizes and shapes.
- Consider the role of the environment within the assessment process; reduce the number of competing distractions on the left-hand side for a person with neglect.

Intervention

- Give a clear explanation of the impairment and its functional consequences to the person and their family.
- Teach compensatory strategies to reduce the impact of the impairment, for example visual scanning techniques, cueing (verbal and visual), learning to check successful task completion, reminders placed in key locations, opportunities for practice.

- Consider interventions for neglect such as limb activation, sensory stimulation and prism adaptation training while acknowledging the experimental nature of these interventions in the absence of robust evidence.
- Take time to understand fully the lived experience of the impairments in order to suggest interventions which hold occupational meaning for the individual.

SUMMARY

1) Body scheme is the mental representation of the position of the parts of the body and the spatial relationship between them. Structural, semantic and lexical representations of body parts are incorporated into the body scheme. The relationship between body scheme disorders and their effect on function has not been clearly defined.

2) There are many different types of agnosia. For example, visuospatial agnosia can be defined as a global impairment of visual and spatial perception which disrupts the interaction of people with objects and with the structure of the physical environment. All everyday tasks become effortful and there is constant strife to regain the person's sense of self.

3) Neglect may occur as information is being inputted from our senses (sensory neglect) or towards the output stage (premotor neglect). People with neglect tend to ignore the side contralateral to the lesion. However, this can vary depending on the amount of data that requires processing and the size of an object in relation to others (relative salience).

4) Assessment and interventions should seek to (a) understand the impact of the impairments on function, (b) restore a person's ability to undertake meaningful activities and occupations within their own environment, and (c) compensate to restore function rather than target the impairment itself.

References

Baas, U., de Haan, D., Grassli, T. *et al.* (2011) Personal neglect – a disorder of body representation? *Neuropsychologia*, **49** (5), 898–905.

Bisiach, E. and Luzatti, C. (1978) Unilateral neglect of representational space. *Cortex*, **14**, 129–133.

Gorgoraptis, N. and Husain, M. (2011) Improving visual neglect after right hemisphere stroke. *Journal of Neurology, Neurosurgery & Psychiatry*, **82**, 1183–1184.

Kerkhoff, G. and Schenk, T. (2012). Rehabilitation of neglect: an update. *Neuropsychologia*, **50**, 1072–1079.

Maddicks, R., Marzillier, S.L. and Parker, G. (2003) Rehabilitation of unilateral neglect in the acute recovery stage: the efficacy of limb activation therapy. *Neuropsychological Rehabilitation*, **13** (3), 391–408.

Robertson, I. and North, N. (1992) Active and passive activation of left limbs: influence on visual and sensory neglect. *Neuropsychologica*, **31**, 293–300.

Robertson, I.H., Hogg, K. and McMillan, T.M. (1998) Rehabilitation of unilateral neglect: improving function by contralesional limb activation. *Neuropsychological Rehabilitation*, **8**, 19–29.

Sirigu, A., Grafman, J., Bressler, K. and Sunderland, T. (1991) Multiple representations contribute to body knowledge processing: evidence from a case of autopagnosia. *Brain*, **114**, 629–642.

Tham, K., Borell, L. and Gustavsson, A. (2000) The discovery of disability: a phenomenological study of unilateral neglect. *American Journal of Occupational Therapy*, **54**, 398–406.

Ting, D.S.J., Pollock, A., Dutton, G.N. *et al.* (2011) Visual neglect following stroke: current concepts and future focus. *Survey of Ophthalmology*, **56** (2), 114–134.

8

Memory

Tess Baird and Linda Maskill

AIMS

1) To outline the lived experience of memory impairments.
2) To debate the different types of memory and neuropsychological models.
3) To explore specific memory processes: registration, retention, retrieval, levels of processing and schema theory.
4) To consider assessment and intervention options.

Introduction

This chapter will introduce the reader to the different types of memory and models for how memory is thought to function. It will consider the evidence base for short-term memory, working memory, the different types of long-term memory and memory processes. Finally, it will focus on the assessment of and treatment options for memory deficits. But to start with, it is important to consider what it is like to live with memory impairment.

The lived experience of impaired memory (adapted from Meltzer 1983)

Driving home from the hospital, I didn't recognise the route but did remember my house when we got there.

   I had to relearn how to use things like the alarm clock or change my razor blade; it often took several trials to get it right because, once my train of thought was interrupted, I had to start from the beginning again. I would get lost when out for a walk in my neighbourhood. I began to feel incompetent and alone, especially as I had also forgotten some of my cultural norms: my traditions and my beliefs.

Neuropsychology for Occupational Therapists: Cognition in Occupational Performance, Fourth Edition.
Edited by Linda Maskill and Stephanie Tempest.
© 2017 John Wiley & Sons Ltd. Published 2017 by John Wiley & Sons Ltd.
Companion Website: www.wiley.com/go/maskill/neuropsychologyOT

Simple recreational activities felt like work: TV plots were hard to follow; some words in my book lost their meaning; conversations could become a trial as I worried about saying the wrong things to people or could not remember much about current events. I became more withdrawn from my family and friends. But then my wife and I started my rehabilitation process.

For patients, I recommend: stay involved in things. Try doing things that are at a lower level than before and keep trying. Write everything down and keep notes on your progress. Don't conceal the memory problem. If something pops into your mind when in conversation – say it, as it is often correct.

For therapists, I recommend: avoiding complicated sentences; minimise distractions; review goals jointly; ask the patient to review and repeat instructions; find things he is competent at; do not deny the memory problems; remember the family – without my wife and daughter I'm not sure how much rehabilitation would have taken place.

The lived experience of impaired memory highlights the links between keeping something in mind, recalling information and executing future actions. It also provides us with an insight of the impact on day-to-day life. Memory is important for our sense of self; it is a culture-specific system and is modified over time by using recall of past experiences to deal with situations in the present (Sternberg 1999).

Classic case studies tell us that memory involves more than one part of the brain (e.g. Milner 1966; Squire 2009). There are individuals who are unable to recall events (impaired declarative memory) but have retained learned motor skills (intact procedural memory). Therefore, no two people with memory loss will present the same. Indeed, global amnesia is very rare. We will start by discussing our understanding of short-term memory (STM).

Short-Term Memory

First, we will consider the different modalities for short-term memory (e.g. verbal and visual STM) and then develop this understanding into a working memory system.

Short-term memory refers to 'the retention of small amounts of information tested over a few seconds' (Baddeley *et al.* 2010) or after a short delay, and can be divided into verbal STM and visual STM. Short-term memory has a limited capacity and retains information over a period of seconds or minutes.

Verbal STM

The presence of a STM store was first shown by experiments which recorded the free recall of numbers, words or pictures.

A quick measure of STM is the digit span test. A sequence of numbers is read out at one digit per second and the person is asked to repeat them back in the same order. The number of digits in the sequence is increased by one digit in each trial. The digit span is the largest number of digits you can get right in one trial.

Miller (1956) suggested that capacity for remembering was not due to the number of items to be recalled but by the number of chunks. Chunking is linked to the natural phrasing we have in language, with it being easier to remember numbers often linked in triplets (Wicklegrne 1964) rather than a long line of single digits. For example 983 – 462 – 175 is easier to remember than 983462175.

Interestingly, STM is relatively well preserved with age. Parkinson *et al.* (1985) demonstrated a slight reduction in digit span dropping from 6.6 to 5.8 over the course of an adult life. It should be noted that these tests only explore some component functions of the short-term memory system.

The predominant features of verbal STM include a reduction in ability to recall information when words sound similar (Conrad 1964), when words are longer or when there is a concurrent distraction (Baddeley *et al.* 2010). This evidence, based in auditory processing, supports Baddeley and Hitch's phonological loop theory (1974) which will be discussed later.

Clinically, working out when recall of information for STM breaks down is useful to help with how information is presented to people. As Glanzer (1972) highlighted, performance on such recall tasks can be enhanced through slower presentation, familiarity of words and highly visual words.

Visual STM

Visual STM can be divided into visual and spatial memory components for experimental and theoretical purposes. However, in real life these two systems work together, creating visuospatial memory.

Short-term memory for spatial locations, such as the positioning of a door in the dark in a new environment, appears to decline over a 30-second period (Thomson 1983). Memory for objects (Vogel *et al.* 2001) seems to be around four items. However, visual STM does not have the extent of experimental evidence base that has been developed for verbal STM.

Working Memory

Short-term memory was originally described as a temporary memory store of a small amount of information to hold it in mind for further analysis before entering the permanent long-term store. Studies of short-term memory in the 1970s, by Baddeley and Hitch, led to the expansion of the structure of STM into a more active working memory system. The term 'working memory' refers to a brain system that provides temporary storage and manipulation of the information necessary for such complex cognitive tasks as language comprehension, learning and reasoning (Baddeley *et al.* 2010). There remains much debate and confusion regarding the differences between short-term and working memory but, in brief, it is considered that working memory involves the manipulation or use of short-term memories.

There are two sources of information entering working memory: one is from incoming sensory memory and the other is from long-term memory. In memory recall, information stored in long-term memory is transferred back into working memory for interpretation of the incoming information. Working memory acts like a workbench, where verbal, visual and spatial information of both new and old memories is manipulated and integrated over a short period of time before passing on to long-term memory and to other cognitive systems. Subsequently, Craik and Lockhart (1972) argued that it was the depth of processing which supported learning rather than the amount of time registered in short-term storage.

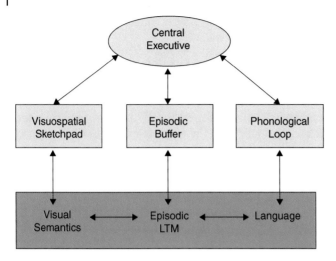

Figure 8.1 Multicomponent working memory model. Source: Baddeley (2000). Reproduced with permission of Elsevier.

Baddeley and Hitch's multicomponent model of working memory (1974) draws upon a wealth of experimental and neuropsychological studies and has stood the test of time in relation to new available evidence. Updated by Baddeley in 2000, the multicomponent model has four main components: the phonological loop, the visuospatial sketchpad, the episodic buffer and the central executive (Figure 8.1).

- The *phonological loop* stores speech-based information in a temporary store or 'inner ear'. Items are verbally rehearsed in the same order in the phonological loop before decay or passing on into long-term memory. Baddeley and Hitch (1974) found that the phonological loop was not limited by the number of items it could hold but by the length of time taken to rehearse them. In speaking and reading, several words are held long enough to make sense of the words that follow. Words can enter the phonological store directly from the ear, from the mental rehearsal of written or spoken words and from long-term memory.
- The *visuospatial sketchpad* is a temporary store of visual and spatial information entering the brain from the eye. This 'inner eye' component of working memory holds information that cannot be rehearsed verbally, such as size, shape, colour and distance, for a short time. The sketchpad is also used to inspect and manipulate visual images entering from long-term memory. If we search for lost keys, visuospatial images at possible locations are manipulated like 'snapshots' and compared with retrieved information from long-term memory. A spatial awareness task can be affected by visual imagery and vice versa. This suggests that these are similar but intertwined systems (Baddeley *et al.* 2010). The visuospatial sketchpad is thought to often combine with the phonological loop to enhance performance. Hatano and Osawa (1983) described how Japanese experts in mental calculation used visual images of the abacus to help them perform complex maths.
- The *episodic buffer* is another component of working memory; it integrates all the processing in working memory, from the phonological loop, the visuospatial sketchpad and long-term memory. This component fills the gap in the general storage of visual and sound-based items into a single episode. For example, the episodic buffer

integrates the visual images of people with their speech when we are watching TV. Baddeley (2007) has also linked the important role that emotion has on memory to the episodic buffer.

- The *central executive* directs and controls the processing in the other components of working memory by the allocation of attention to each one. The central executive is particularly important when the cognitive demands of a task are high, or when we are doing two or more things at a time. The central executive has two operational modes. First, one which is based on automatic actions, often linked to habits, for example an experienced car driver who drives home with no real recall of how he got there. Second, there is the supervisory attentional system which intervenes when problem-solving and consequent actions are required, which are more closely linked with executive functioning, e.g. driving on a diverted, unfamiliar route. With the central executive having very close links with all areas of attention, it is a key component of effective working memory.

A number of attentional tasks have been linked with memory issues as well, highlighting the interplay of cognitive skills for occupational performance. Robbins *et al.* (1996) compared the effects of differing types of distractions on recalling positions of chess pieces on a chess board. Strayer and Johnson (2001) demonstrated that on a driving simulator, the introduction of speaking on a mobile phone meant the drivers were more likely to miss red lights and were significantly slower at applying the brakes in an emergency situation.

The working memory model offers an account of how the abundance of sensory information continually entering the brain is rehearsed over a brief period of time to organise and associate it into a form that can be passed on to the other components of the cognitive system. Neuroimaging studies have shown that the active brain areas in working memory function are widely distributed anatomically. In a PET scan study of normal subjects performing verbal tasks, the phonological store was localised in the supramarginal gyrus of the left parietal lobe, and the articulatory loop for rehearsal in Broca's area of the frontal lobe (Paulesu *et al.* 1993). In another study involving spatial memory, increased cerebral blood flow was recorded in the right parietal and right pre-frontal cortices (Jonides *et al.* 1993). There is evidence to locate the central executive in the frontal lobe overlapping with the supervisory attention system (see Chapter 10: Executive Functions).

Impairments of Working Memory

People with working memory deficits can function in daily living when tasks do not make major cognitive demands, but find it harder to process information from two or more sources simultaneously and multitask. The components of working memory can be selectively impaired so that some people with brain damage may not be able to recall numbers or words that are heard, but can recall the same information when it is presented visually. Working memory can remain intact when there is severe impairment of long-term memory and vice versa.

Living with Working Memory Deficits

Deficits in working memory affect communication. In speaking, long sentences cannot be held and rehearsed in the phonological loop long enough for understanding. The same problem affects reading. A long article in the newspaper may be difficult to understand, but comprehension is improved when it is divided into short chunks or when accessing news via Twitter feeds. It may be difficult to find the way to the super-market if visual images of landmarks cannot be integrated with retrieved long-term memory of the route. People with working memory deficit can only copy the movements of a therapist when they are done concurrently. If there is a delay before imitation, the visual and verbal input from the therapist is lost.

Doing two things at a time is difficult for many people. This affects parents and carers of young children, when daily living tasks are done whilst monitoring their play. Leisure activities that involve the visual and spatial organisation of items or keeping a score may be difficult.

Long-Term Memory

Long-term memory (LTM) is a system or systems assumed to underpin the ability to store information over long periods of time (Baddeley *et al.* 2010). Long-term memory has unlimited capacity and processes a large variety of information which is constantly updated. Some items from working memory enter LTM where they are processed for meaning and context. In reverse, stored memories in LTM are retrieved into working memory for manipulation and reflection before the relevant response is activated. Figure 8.2 shows how the sensory, working and long-term memory systems interact.

Long-term memory, as shown in Figure 8.2, has been classified into two broad areas: declarative (explicit) and non-declarative (procedural or implicit) memory (Squire 1992). In addition, 'metamemory' has also been identified, which includes source moni-toring, prospective memory and 'knowing what you know' (see Ashcraft and Radvansky 2010). Figure 8.3 summarises these main divisions of LTM function. We will now con-sider these main subdivisions in turn.

Declarative (Explicit) Memory

Declarative memory is the knowledge of people, objects, places and events. It is the memory that allows us to state whether certain facts are true or false. Declarative

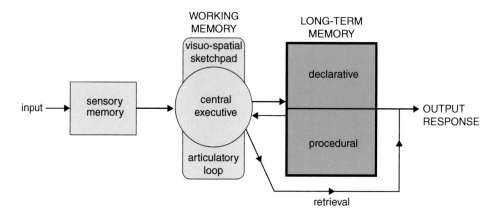

Figure 8.2 The interactions between the three memory systems.

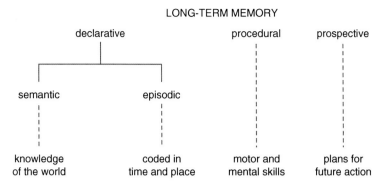

Figure 8.3 The main divisions of long-term memory.

memory can be called 'knowing what'. It is explicit. If we are asked a concrete question, for example 'Where were you born?', we consciously inspect declarative memory to recall the name of the place. Declarative memory has been divided into two main types: semantic and episodic.

- *Semantic memory* relates to knowledge of the world, without reference to how or when information was learnt; you know that Rome is the capital of Italy. Semantic memories are organised by concept and associations into a complex knowledge base and they can be retrieved without context. Semantic memory is referred to as general knowledge of the world but also includes vocabulary (Baddeley *et al.* 2010).
- *Episodic memory* relates to the memories of facts and events in their context. It refers to a particular episode or event in our lives that occurred in a particular time and place. It enables us, for example, to remember a conversation we had half an hour ago with a colleague and recall the person we met on the bus yesterday. Tulving (2002) thinks about this in terms of experiencing some aspect of the original episode to help relive the event to help you plan for future action.

The organisation of semantic knowledge has led to a number of differing theories on how semantic information is stored in our brains. Cree and McRae (2003) suggested that semantic memory is organised through seven different categories: visual motion, visual parts, colour, function, taste, smell and sound. They called this the multiproperty approach and it reflects evidence from neuropsychological and brain imaging studies. However, this approach does not reflect the complexities of everyday life, whereas schema theory seems to offer that option. Schemas are well-integrated chunks of knowledge about the world, events, people or actions. They allow us to form expectations about experiences and are important in reading and listening as they help us fill the gaps, which then improves our understanding of a situation (Sulin and Dooling 1974), and they help us when we are looking at a visual scene (Brewer and Treyens 1981).

Retrieval from episodic memory depends on the ability to recall the relevant contextual information of the time and place that it occurred, and this happens more easily in the same context that it was learnt. Riding on the same bus on another occasion may help us to retrieve knowledge of the person we met on a previous bus journey.

Some clinicians and psychologists have distinguished recent and remote episodic memory (Levy 2001). Recent episodic memory is the ability to remember people, places and daily events that occurred a short time ago and they reflect a person's potential for learning new memories. A person visiting the occupational therapy department develops recent episodic memory of the layout of the rooms and the names of the staff. Recent episodic memory is the least durable of all types of memory and its impairment is often the first sign of memory loss. Older adults often experience lapses of recent episodic memory – for example, they may go upstairs and then not remember why, or they may not be able to find the right glasses to read the newspaper. Younger people may do the same, particularly when they are stressed.

Remote episodic memory of events that occurred years before is more durable. Places and names associated with a person's family history, such as birthdays, weddings and births, from many years before form the remote episodic memory. Memories of these events are often retained in great detail, while at the same time recent episodic memory is impaired. Some people with severe loss of cognitive function do retain remote episodic memory going back to early childhood, hence the value of reminiscence in therapy sessions for these people.

Episodic memory is thought of as the capacity to remember specific events, which requires three components. First, it requires the ability to encode the particular experience to be able to separate it from other similar events. Next, this experience needs to be coded in a form that can be recalled and finally, we need the ability to search and retrieve the event.

The evidence suggests that episodic memory needs to encode a particular experience but separate it from similar events. However, knowledge of a similar event that happened previously can influence recall of the later event, as can the meaning of the words used to elicit that recall. An example of this is given below where we consider the integrated functioning of memory processes.

Episodic Versus Semantic?

Semantic and episodic aspects interact in everyday memory. This makes research into one or the other challenging, as there is a very close link between events we experience and our knowledge of the world. Tulving (2002) suggested that semantic and episodic memory are interlinked, as often semantic memories are made up of a series of episodic ones. Knowledge that began as episodic becomes generalised into semantic memory over time. When you meet someone for the first time, the event is stored in episodic memory. After a time, knowledge about the person, for example colour of eyes and hair, is stored in semantic memory. This example illustrates the parallel storage of items in different memory systems.

Support for the distinction between semantic and episodic memory comes from studies of people with memory loss who demonstrate impairment of episodic memory but have no difficulty in the recall of the semantic knowledge they learned before onset. Spiers *et al.* (2001), in their review of 147 amnesic case reports, found that the majority of patients suffered with issues around episodic memory but only a few for semantic memory. So although closely linked, they are distinct and separate systems.

Maguire *et al.*'s (1997) study of London taxi drivers demonstrated that learning large amounts of semantic and episodic information (the Knowledge – a detailed store of information about places and routes in London) led to volume changes in the hippocampus, and was also related to length of time as a taxi driver – the longer the time, the greater the change.

Autobiographical Memory

Conway (2005) described autobiographical memory as 'a system that retains knowledge concerning the experienced self, the me'. It is memory across the lifespan for both certain events and self-related information and therefore comprises episodic and semantic memory combining into a meaningful personal history.

Williams *et al.* (2008) propose four different types of autobiographical memory. First, 'biographical' or 'personal', for example who you are or where you were born. Second, there is the concept of how authentic the memories are, dividing into 'copies' or 'reconstructions'. Copies are vivid memories of an experience whereas reconstructions are memories that are rebuilt to incorporate new information or interpretations made in hindsight. Third is the 'specific' or 'generic' type, where the key is the depth of detail. Finally, there is the concept of 'field' or 'observer', focusing on whether the event happened to you or you were an observer in the event recalled.

Retrograde amnesia often leads to a loss of episodic memories for specific events and semantic autobiographical knowledge such as remembering school friends' names. De Renzi *et al.* (1987) demonstrated in a single case report that this is not always the case. The lady in question had little or no recall for public events or names of famous people of the time but had excellent recall for her personal life story. Whereas Dalla Barba *et al.* (1990) reported an incident of a gentleman with Korsakoff's syndrome for whom the reverse was true.

Confabulation is an example of a disrupted autobiographical memory. It is where information is false but not intentionally misleading. Baddeley and Wilson (1988) described the case of RR, who suffered significant frontal lobe damage after a car crash. He gave a detailed and plausible description of the events post car crash, although it was reported that he was unconscious for this whole time period.

Confabulation is typically found in patients suffering from executive dysfunction due to frontal lobe damage. It is thought to disturb autobiographical memory in two ways. First, due to issues with recall of the correct cues to help with the memory and second, implausible information is often accepted by those with frontal lobe damage and then elaborated on.

Conway *et al.* (2003) used electroencephalography in their study of autobiographical memory. They suggested that in the early stages of the task, the prefrontal cortex was activated and then latterly the occipital and temporal lobes. This evidence links nicely with Greenberg and Rubin (2003) who noted that patients who had difficulties with autobiographical memory often had damage in areas of the brain associated with visualisation. This suggests that the frontal lobes are important for evoking the memory and then the visual imagery of the event comes second.

In their meta-analysis on the functional neuroanatomy of autobiographical memory, Svoboda *et al.* (2006) highlighted the difference on a neuroanatomical basis between the episodic and semantic aspects of autobiographical memory. Greenberg *et al.* (2005), using fMRI, found that autobiographical retrieval was linked to the amygdala, classically related to emotions. The hippocampus supported episodic memory and semantic retrieval resulted in activation of the left frontal lobes.

Procedural (Implicit or Non-Declarative) Memory

Procedural (implicit or non-declarative) memory is about retrieval of information through performance rather than conscious recall or recognition. Procedural memory has been predominantly studied through amnesic patients whose rate of learning procedural information seems to be the same as normal individuals. Case studies have also demonstrated that people with severe LTM impairment (not being able to retain episodic or semantic memories) can retain procedural memories. In the classic case of patient HM (Squire 2009), he was able to acquire and retain a learned motor skill (mirror tracing) over time, even though he had no episodic memory of the sessions in which he practised the skill.

In a study of classical conditioning, Weiskrantz and Warrington (1979) demonstrated that amnesic individuals would, after a tone, blink in preparation for a puff of air directed into their eye, but could not remember that this would be going to happen.

Warrington and Weiskrantz (1968) demonstrated that word learning can be pre-served in amnesic individuals. When a list of words was presented including the word 'metal', and after a delay the participants were then asked to guess a word starting with 'm,e,...', they would guess the word 'metal' more frequently than would be expected if no prior exposure had occurred. This suggests that some form of encoding is happening. This is an example of priming where the presentation of an item influences the processing of the next item.

Case study (Wilson and Wearing 1995)

CW suffered severe memory loss following the viral infection herpes simplex encephalitis. Brain scans showed that his left and part of his right temporal lobes had been destroyed. He had previously had a successful career as a professional musician. He developed severe amnesia for the time following the onset of his illness and was unable to acquire new memories. Also, he could not remember any episodes from his life before onset except a few facts from his childhood. He could recognise his wife but he had difficulty in recognising common objects and could not remember what had happened a few minutes before. Any conversation he had with another person was immediately forgotten. If he went out, he got lost and could not find his way back. In spite of CW's severe memory loss, his procedural memory was spared so that he could still play the piano and sight-read music with great skill.

Everyday routine tasks are mostly automatic and depend on implicit procedural memory, for example making a cup of tea, following one's morning routine for getting up or driving a car. People with dementia, even if severe, may retain knowledge of how to do familiar well-practised action sequences and tasks, although these may be triggered or occur inappropriately, and self-monitoring of the performance is deficient. Therapeutic approaches in dementia care may make use of cueing or priming, to help elicit procedural memories, to aid in daily tasks like dressing or engagement in familiar and previously enjoyed activities.

Metamemory

Metamemory is a concept concerning LTM functions that relate to a person's use and manipulation of memory. It has been defined as 'the ability to assess when you've learned something, that you need to remember something in the future'

(Ashcraft and Radvansky 2010, p. 291). It also incorporates the ability to monitor the source of a memory (was it a real event or did you just think it?), and 'knowing what you know'. Metamemory therefore can be considered a set of functions that overlap and require close integration with executive functioning i.e with our self-awareness, ability to evaluate information and monitor ourselves, in order to produce appropriate, timely and meaningful behaviours in context.

Prospective Memory

Prospective memory is about remembering to do things in the future, recalling conscious decisions and plans in order to carry them through and act. It is therefore associated with the executive functions of the frontal cortex. Prospective memory has been further divided into two categories: event based and time based. Event-based memory is where some event (e.g. seeing your local shop) provides the cue to create an action (e.g. buying some milk). Time-based memory is where the actual time acts as a cue to trigger an action. Hence, in non-routine activities, which have to be remembered occasionally, time-based prospective memory is needed to activate the plan at the right time. Where there is an external cue to activate the plan, event-based memory prompts you to go into the shop.

In the absence of a cue, the attention demands in working memory may affect the success or failure of prospective memory. We forget to make an important phone call on a busy day when there are many demands on our attention.

There are elements of retrospective memory in the performance of future actions; for example, remembering to take medication at intervals in the day is prospective, while remembering how many and the colour of each tablet is retrospective. Ageing impacts more on retrospective than prospective memory (Henry *et al.* 2004) with event-based prospective memory tasks being particularly difficult when distractions are introduced. However, in prospective memory tasks where the focus is on more practical situations, for example phone numbers and appointments, older people do better than their younger counterparts.

The success of compensatory strategies to improve prospective memory depends largely on the development of self-awareness (Fleming *et al.* 2005). The person with memory loss needs to acknowledge the existence of problems and impaired self-aware-ness needs to be addressed before any external aids are introduced. Once self-awareness is established, there is motivation to use organisational devices over an extended period.

Prospective memory failure is seen frequently in people recovering from traumatic brain injury. Fish *et al.* (2010, p. 171) stated that prospective memory should be viewed as 'a type of functional goal that makes demands on our capacity rather than an isolated form of memory'. Impairments are most likely to compromise daily living skills through forgetting important tasks and being unable to use strategies effectively.

Although theories of prospective memory point to attention as one of its primary limiting factors (Smith and Bayen 2005), Fish reminds us that it is the implementation of strategies linked to executive functioning which affects day-to-day performance on this issue (Fish *et al.* 2008).

Source Monitoring

Source monitoring refers to our ability to remember where information has come from. This is important for us to differentiate between what has actually happened, or is fact, from what we might have imagined or only thought about. For students, a critical example of the value of source monitoring is in ensuring academic sources are appropriately identified and acknowledged. Failure of source monitoring may result in inadvertent plagiarism if a student has read something but, in going on to develop their own views about it, fails to recall that the original idea was not their own. Source monitoring also functions in being able to recall whether or not you have actually done something that you normally do every day or several times a day, such as when you cannot recall if you locked the door on your way to work. It enables us to know whether we have done something or just thought about it (Ashcraft and Radvansky 2010).

Most people experience the consequences of a failure of source monitoring at some point in their daily lives. It can have potentially serious consequences, and can cause distress for those who, for example, experience hallucinations or delusions (being unable to differentiate reality from internally generated experiences) or people with deficits of declarative memory who cannot recall where or when they gained certain information or experience.

Activity

Answer the following questions.

- Who was the British Prime Minister who succeeded Tony Blair?
- How many teachers can you name from your primary and secondary school days?
- Do you remember learning to ride a bike?
- If you gave a detailed set of instructions to someone who could not ride a bike, would he or she be able to do it? If not, why not?
- If you received a text from your mum asking you to call her in an hour, tomorrow morning or next Wednesday, what factors will determine if you will do it?

Discuss the memory systems related to these questions.

So far in this chapter, we have explored the lived experience of memory impairment and considered different types of memory. Next we need to explore the specific processes that occur as we seek to use our memory to register, retain, retrieve and process information.

Memory Processes

Neisser (1967) took the computer as an analogy and argued that human memory could be regarded as being composed of one or more storage systems. He proposed that all memory systems require three separate but interacting components which we will explore in turn next.

- Registration or encoding at the time of learning
- Retention or storage over time
- Retrieval and recall of information when it is required

Malia and Brannagan (2005) rightly added attention to the beginning of the process as it acts as a prerequisite for all cognitive processes.

Registration has been explored by manipulating the features and context of the information that is learnt, and testing the subsequent recall to see what factors are most important. Information that is elaborated and processed with meaning at the time of registration increases the likelihood of later retrieval. Some of the strategies we use to improve our memory use elaboration and association, for example retracing our steps to remember where we put something or associating the name of a person with visual imagery of his/her unique features.

Retention is a dynamic process. Stored knowledge is modified and updated by new information entering from working memory over time. Once an item has been registered in memory, subsequent forgetting could be the result of decay over time or it could be due to interference by later learning. Recall of an event depends upon the number of similar events that have occurred, rather than the time that has elapsed, suggesting that new memories interfere with knowledge of past experience (see further discussion below). Consolidation involves the rehearsal of information so it is not lost.

Retrieval involves active cognitive processing. There are two types of retrieval. Recall is a search process followed by a decision process, while recognition only involves the decision process, so that recognition is easier than recall. Retrieval is affected by the context, and items are more likely to be retrieved in the same environment as they were learnt. Attention to cues is thought to be important for effective retrieval. Fernandes and Moscovitch (2003) demonstrated that retrieval can be affected as much as 30–50% by dual tasking. This may be important to consider in terms of the environment when testing a person's ability to retrieve information from memory.

Cues have to be relevant to the memory for which we are searching. For a cue to be useful, it needs to be present at encoding (Tulving and Thompson 1973). Context cues provide additional support at the encoding stage – the memory of seeing a star fruit in a market on holiday is much stronger than seeing the word written on a page. This suggests why new learning in a hospital occupational therapy department may not generalise to the home environment. Similarly, retrieval can fail if the cues are relevant but not strong enough to link towards the target memory.

Recall is improved when there are emotions attached to the memory (Blaney 1986). For example, it is easier to recall happier memories when you are in a good mood and vice versa.

External cueing is an important aid to retrieval of items or events from memory. Recall of the name of a person is improved if it is cued by the first letter or other information about the person. Recognition of the person from a group of names or photographs will assist successful retrieval. We are all familiar with the 'tip of the tongue' phenomenon, when we know an item is in memory but we cannot retrieve it. One explanation is that the current processing does not match the stored information and fails to cue the memory. Some implicit retrieval may occur which is activated at a later time and recall is then achieved.

Levels of Processing

Early studies of memory in the 1970s resulted in the levels of processing theory, which proposed that the depth to which information is encoded determines what is stored in LTM. Information is processed at different levels ranging from shallow, for example detecting specific letters in a word, to deep semantic analysis for meaning.

In a study of the recall of words, Craik and Tulving (1975) presented a list of 60 words to three different groups of subjects. Each group was given an additional question which oriented their perceptual processing to a particular level. The structural group was asked a question about the physical characteristics of the word, 'Is the word in capital letters?'. The acoustic group was asked to process the sound of the word, 'Does the word rhyme with…?'. The semantic group was asked, 'Does the word fit into a given sentence?'. The results showed that success in retrieval of the words was greatest in the group who performed deeper semantic processing. The effect of processing depth was not only shown for verbal items but also for visual recognition. Scores were higher for face recognition when the subjects had reported the pleasantness of each face compared with reporting the structural features of each face.

The levels of processing theory was originally criticised for its inadequate definition of what is meant by the depth of processing. A later model of memory proposed parallel encoding of structural, acoustic and semantic information so that elaboration of the memory trace occurred in the three domains simultaneously. This more elaborated memory trace may create additional routes for retrieval of the item. Another explanation is that extensive input processing produces a more distinctive memory trace that is unique amongst other items in storage. It is possible that *elaboration* and *distinctiveness* operate together to facilitate retrieval in memory.

We can use different levels of processing as an internal strategy to improve our own memory. We are often confronted by a group situation with people we have not met before where we need to learn their names. Our success in remembering their names is increased if we direct our perceptual processing of each person in several ways, for example the position in the group where the person is sitting, their physical features and their behavioural characteristics. In this way, we may remember the name of Peter as the one with the beard, who sits at the back of the group and asks a lot of questions. Other memory aids based on the level of processing are the use of mnemonics, association and grouping. The number of PIN numbers and passwords we have to remember is increasing, so we need to resort to these methods for making recall easier, for example by using the initials and house numbers of our friends and family.

Memory for past events is often affected by our emotional state at the time, for example the details about our first day at school. More extreme examples leave detailed memories of all the contextual features at the time. An example was hearing the news of the terrorist bombing on the London Underground in 2005. Most people in London can remember when and where they were, and who told them about the incident. Such events, known as *flashbulb memories*, may have unique registration in memory but the frequent rehearsal and retelling of the event may account for the detail of the recall rather than a special mechanism.

Schema Theory

Everyday memory involves the organisation and storage of large amounts of complex knowledge. Our success in the recall is variable. Some of our experiences are remembered, others are not, and also the recall is sometimes inaccurate or incomplete. One of the first psychologists to address the organisation of knowledge was Bartlett in the 1930s. He presented English subjects with a North American folk tale which was completely unfamiliar to Western culture. When the subjects were later asked to recall the tale, their accounts were reconstructed to make more sense in terms of their own

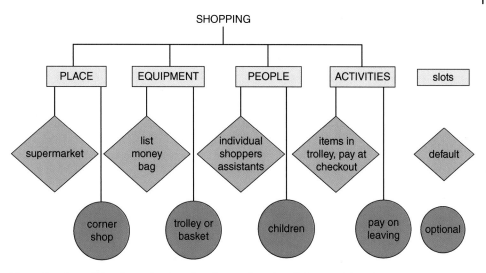

Figure 8.4 A possible schema for shopping. Source: Based on Cohen *et al.* (1993).

experience. He suggested that top-down processing of the new information was incorporated into prestored knowledge to fit with prior expectations (Bartlett 1932).

Bartlett introduced the term *schema*, which is a packet of information stored in memory representing general knowledge. Schemas are modified, updated over time and transformed into a typical form. Generalisations are made from our own experience. Schemas can be simple or complex and they can relate to objects, situations, events or actions. A representation of simple knowledge would be a schema for the letter 'A'. A complex schema would be the knowledge related to a visit to the cinema. This complex schema may have a set of subschemas which include buying the ticket, finding a seat and eating popcorn. The cinema schema may be part of a larger schema for 'outings', together with a visit to the theatre or a football match.

A possible schema for 'shopping' is given in Figure 8.4. The schema specifies the knowledge that is common to all shopping: place, equipment, people and actions, known as the slots. Each slot contains the concepts or actions related to it, with default values if information is not available. The optional values are acquired from particular episodes of shopping.

The way our knowledge is organised influences memory in several ways. Schemas guide the selection of what is encoded at the time of registration. Recall of the schema for a particular visit to the cinema may have ignored what you were wearing at the time, while including the price of the ticket. Schemas transform information from the specific to the general and this can lead to recall of the common features of an experience rather than the details of a particular episode. Top-down processing explains the errors that are made in reporting events we experience when we remember what we expected to see rather than what we actually saw.

Schema theory does account for many of the features of everyday memory and provides a framework for the way that stored complex knowledge incorporates different types of memory. It has been criticised as being too simple and overemphasising the inaccuracy of memory. It does not explain how some complex events are recalled with great detail.

Integrated Functioning of Memory Processes

An example can be used to illustrate how the various components of memory and memory processes work together. Episodic memory requires the ability to remember specific events and to be able to separate them from other similar events. Evidence comes from the work of Sulin and Dooling (1974). They presented two groups of participants with the same information about 'a ruthless and uncontrollable dictator'. The first group were told this person's name was Gerald Martin and the second group were told it was Adolf Hitler. Both groups showed similar recall of the information five minutes after reading the passage. However, a week after the event, their schematic knowledge of Adolf Hitler had influenced their recall, resulting in the Hitler group recalling information that had not been included in the original passage. This helps us understand that knowledge influences memory, that the meaning of words can influence our recall, the role of schemas and that accuracy of source monitoring can be undermined by the interference of previous memories.

Impairment of Long-Term Memory

Memory is affected in many neurological conditions: traumatic brain injury, stroke, viral infection, degenerative disorders, cumulative brain damage in some boxers and footballers, and anoxia in cardiac surgery. There is also psychogenic amnesia, which occurs after ECT and in depression.

Visual memory is more likely to be impaired in right brain-damaged people and verbal memory in left brain damage. The relative impairment of visual and verbal memory affects both the adaptation of the person's environment and the choice of effective cues to be used by the therapist. The overall memory capacity may be reduced. One way to assess this is by reading a short story to the memory-impaired person who is then asked to select picture cards which illustrate it. This simple test can reveal the features of the person's memory function from the observation of the type and position of omissions and errors. It also gives an indication of problems with sequencing as well as total memory capacity.

Semantic and procedural memory are both durable and minimally affected by ageing. Marked changes with age may occur, however, in recent episodic memory. There is difficulty in processing newly acquired information which is not related to a person's stored semantic knowledge. This is experienced as forgetting the names of people, items of shopping and the location of objects. Older adults often report a loss of STM but their problem really relates to recent episodic memory (Levy 2001).

Amnesia

Amnesia is the term used to describe a severe impairment of LTM in the presence of relatively preserved cognitive abilities. The term *anterograde amnesia* (AA) refers to the impairment of memory for events and experiences since the onset. *Retrograde amnesia* (RA) refers to loss of memory for the period before the onset. This distinction into two types gives the means to decide whether the problem is related to learning new material

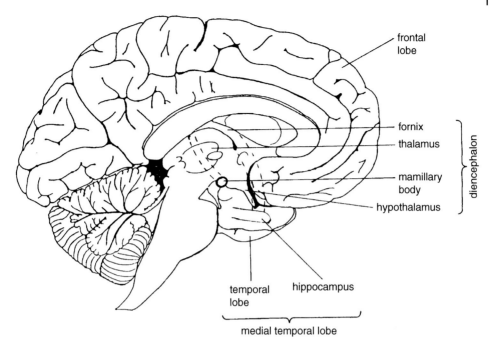

Figure 8.5 Sagittal section of the brain showing the position of the diencephalon and the medial temporal lobe.

or inability to retrieve past information. If the amnesia is a learning disorder, the person will have AA but no RA. If the cause of amnesia is a retrieval deficit, the memory loss will be both anterograde and retrograde. In reality, amnesics vary a great deal in the relative severity of anterograde and retrograde loss.

There is some evidence that the underlying causes of amnesia are linked to damage in two different areas of the brain (Figure 8.5).

- The *diencephalon* is a subcortical area lying at the base of the forebrain. It includes the dorsomedial nucleus of the thalamus and the mamillary bodies. This brain area is associated with both anterograde and retrograde amnesia due to decay in storage of memory traces and retrieval problems. Diencephalic amnesia occurs as a result of chronic alcoholism and the associated thiamine deficiency. In Korsakoff's amnesia, the frontal lobe is also typically damaged.
- The *medial temporal lobe* and *hippocampus* are associated with severe anterograde loss, characterised by inability to learn and store new material. Temporal lobe amnesia occurs after severe temporal lobe damage due to viral encephalitis and progressive atrophy in Alzheimer's disease. PET scan studies have shown that the hippocampus plays an important role in episodic memory. Some of the features of temporal lobe amnesia are described in the case study from Wilson and Wearing (1995) given in the section on procedural memory. Further exploration of all memory disorders can be found in Baddeley *et al.* (2002).

Confabulation

Confabulation is the falsification of memory associated with amnesia. It has been called 'honest lying'. *Spontaneous confabulation* is unprovoked and the person may act according to a false memory. There is a failure to suppress currently irrelevant memories which intrude on the present time so that actions or speech are put in the wrong context. For example, an amnesic person who was a former executive regularly asked to leave the hospital ward to go to a meeting. *Non-spontaneous confabulations* are provoked in answer to a question. Incorrect information, though plausible, is given in response to questions such as 'Have you seen this before?' or 'How many children do you have?'. Both the details and the context of a memory are confused, and the relationship of events in time is disrupted. Confabulation is not a simple loss of memories and it coincides with a loss of insight.

Retrieval in normal memory requires the development of a strategy to activate stored knowledge with particular time and space dimensions, as well as verification of its plausibility and consistency with other information. If there is a loss of these checking procedures, there is no insight. Confabulation most frequently occurs in people with frontal lobe lesions. The common features of processing and the anatomical location suggest that confabulation may be a memory impairment with an overlay of executive dysfunction (see Chapter 10). It might therefore be considered to be a failure of metamemory functions.

Living with Long-Term Memory Deficits

The inability to recognise objects, faces and landmarks can be the result of LTM loss. In daily living, familiar articles in a home setting are the most likely to be recognised. The memory-impaired person may place articles in unusual positions in the house, for example a kitchen utensil on a table in the bathroom. Daily routines are either not activated at the right time or not activated at all. People with severe loss of prospective memory are not able to live independently. Memory for former daily routines and appointments may be intact, except when they involve information or words that are no longer in semantic memory. The timetable for daily or weekly events may not be recalled, for example when to put out the bin. Parents organising young children need to remember which day a child goes swimming or needs to take dinner money. Personal or family safety may be compromised if the person cannot remember whether the door was locked or the gas was turned off on the cooker. Friends may be upset when social engagements are forgotten.

Memory dysfunction can lead to loss of identity and independence. The phrase 'we are what we remember' expresses clearly the importance of memories of the past to give us a sense of self. People, places and objects, as well as the events we have experienced, are part of autobiographical memory. A vase on a shelf or a postcard in a drawer can vividly retrieve the memory of a holiday in the distant past with all the associated people and events. When this memory has gone, the sense of loss for the family and friends, as well as the person, is great. Social interaction with family and friends is difficult when the person cannot talk about the events they have enjoyed together in the past and this may lead to a loss of self-esteem. The identification of a spared work or leisure skill may restore self-esteem and provide motivation for further memory training.

Watching TV, visiting the cinema and reading the newspaper cannot be enjoyed if the storyline cannot be followed. Sport enthusiasts cannot remember what happened in the last game. Spared procedural memory retains the ability to perform sporting activities learnt in the past, although memory aids are needed for the parts of the activity that rely on semantic memory, for example scoring.

Memory loss may have minimum effect on some people who are well supported by family and carers. For others, the loss may have widespread effects on daily living, social interaction, leisure pursuits and employment. After brain damage, some people deny that they have a memory problem because their new environment makes few demands on memory. In degenerative conditions, the deterioration of memory may be gradual and difficult to separate from other cognitive changes.

Suggestions for Assessment and Intervention

Assessment

There are a large number of assessments that can be used for assessing memory. Most tasks include recognition and recall components which can then be used to assess memory processes. Standardised measures, for example those listed below, were previously recommended by the Intercollegiate Stroke Working Party (Intercollegiate Stroke Working Party 2012, p. 118):

- Rivermead Behavioural Memory Test-3 (Wilson *et al.* 2008)
- Doors and People (Baddeley *et al.* 1994)
- Wechsler Memory Test – WMS-IV (Wechsler 2008)
- Repeatable Battery for the Assessment of Neuropsychological Status (RBANS) (Randolph 1998)
- Addenbrookes Cognitive Examination – ACE-R (Mioshi *et al.* 2006)
- Mini-Mental State Examination (MMSE) (Folstein *et al.* 1975).

While objective techniques provide the most reliable assessments of memory, self-report questionnaires can also provide valuable information about the extent to which participants experience their memory as being impaired. Common questionnaires include:

- Everyday Memory Questionnaire (Sunderland *et al.* 1984, revised Royle and Lincoln 2008)
- Prospective and Retrospective Memory Questionnaire (PRMQ) (Smith *et al.* 2000)
- Memory Self Efficacy Scale (Berry and West 1993).

As discussed in Chapter 2, common everyday tasks can be used to screen in an informal but systematic way for cognitive deficits, and can be used by all members of the multidisciplinary team. For informal memory assessment, being specific with instructions around a task will help with identifying where the memory processes are breaking down.

Short-Term Memory

Give brief task instructions, for example 'I want to see if you can get from the bed to the chair, can you repeat that back to me so I know you have understood?'.

- If the person can't repeat them straight back to you then assess their attention further.
- If they can, move on to assessment of encoding.

Encoding

Give more details – the steps involved in the task, for example 'To do this safely, you need to 1. move your bottom forward, 2. check your feet, 3. bring your shoulders forward to hold onto the chair and 4. stand up... Can you repeat that back to me so I know you have understood?'.

- If the person can't recall the steps but can do with a prompt, for example 'Should you check your feet or reach for the chair first?', then they can potentially encode but are having problems with retrieval of this information.

Consolidation and Storage

Give the details of the task, ask them to repeat, create delay by talking about something else, then prompt to do task, for example 'To do this safely you need to 1. move your bottom forward, 2. check your feet, 3. bring your shoulders forward to hold onto the chair and 4. stand up... Can you repeat that back to me so I know you have understood?'

- Engage the person in a different conversation or see if they can recall the steps in the next session – do they carry over the information: 'Can you now remember the steps to getting off the bed?'.

Retrieval

Ask them to show what they did in the last session, for example 'Show me the steps for getting off the bed'.

- If they can, then they can encode, consolidate and retrieve on a functional level.
- If they cannot, make sure you evaluate the number and type of prompts you give.

Intervention

Memory rehabilitation is concerned with the achievement of individual goals rather than improvement or restoration of the specific cognitive functions, and within a holistic framework (Wilson 2003). As with interventions for other cognitive impairments, rehabilitation is effective in helping patients learn and apply compensations for residual memory limitations, although several trials indicate some intervention may directly improve underlying functions. However, there is still limited evidence regarding improvements at the level of functional activities, participation or life satisfaction after cognitive rehabilitation. Cognitive rehabilitation is effective during the postacute period but also even many years after the initial injury (Cicerone *et al.* 2005).

Individuals with memory problems should:

- have nursing and therapy sessions altered to capitalise on preserved abilities
- be taught approaches that help them to encode, store and retrieve new information, for example, spaced retrieval (increasing time intervals between review of information) or deep encoding of material (emphasising semantic features)
- have therapy delivered in an environment that is as similar to the usual environment for that patient as possible (Intercollegiate Stroke Working Party 2016).

The specific approaches, methods and techniques employed will depend upon the individual needs, impairments and preserved abilities of the person, but could include education, remediation or compensation.

- *Education* – improving individuals' understanding of their own memory difficulties and developing awareness of how their impairments impact on their everyday life are essential aspects of memory rehabilitation (Burke *et al.* 1994).
- *Remediation* – people with dementia and their caregivers are often advised that 'mental exercise' may be helpful in slowing down the decline in memory and thinking experienced by many people with dementia. Cognitive stimulation involves a wide range of activities, often in a group, that aim to stimulate thinking and memory generally, including discussion of past and present events and topics of interest, word games, puzzles, music and practical activities such as baking or indoor gardening.
- *Compensation* – internal or external strategies are effective in improving recall performance for people with mild memory impairment, for example a paging system (Wilson *et al.* 2005). Advances in the technology of smartphones have provided opportunities to use strategies within an everyday context, for example setting reminders.

Intensity, Feedback and the Structure of Practice

Frequency and intensity are critical in improving memory performance (Hildebrandt *et al.* 2011). Generally, breaking practice up into a number of shorter sessions (distributed practice) is better than fewer but longer sessions (mass practice).

Feedback is a crucial part of learning, so if feedback is not given, errors tend to persist (Pashler *et al.* 2007). If feedback is given then errors are less likely to be made and retained. This is fundamental understanding around the principles of errorless learning (EL).

Errorless Learning

Clare and Jones (2008) identified a number of characteristics of tasks that are likely to work well using EL methods. In relation to the task, it should ideally involve one cognitive domain and a single component of behaviour, or the task can be broken down into specific steps. The task or task steps should be concrete. The task needs to be relevant to the individual and pretraining can be undertaken to improve performance (Kalla *et al.* 2001). Support for the benefits of EL compared to trial-and-error or error-full (EF) learning conditions for people with memory impairments comes from a number of studies of people with brain injury (Baddeley and Wilson 1994; Page *et al.* 2006). However, people with early-stage Alzheimer's disease appear to do equally well with EL and EF methods (Clare and Jones 2008). It can be hypothesised that people with less severe impairment in explicit memory who retain the ability to monitor and detect errors, and to update knowledge of their performance on the basis of feedback (Morris and Hannesdottir 2004), may not require error elimination or error reduction, while people with more severe impairments in explicit memory and difficulties in monitoring and detecting performance errors might require EL methods in order to demonstrate effective learning.

SUMMARY

1) Working memory theory is an account of how verbal and visuospatial information from the sensory store is held for a short time, while some active processing for meaning occurs, before passing on to long-term memory. Verbal (speech-based) items are rehearsed in the phonological loop. Attention is allocated between the visual and verbal components by a central executive. Items from visual and verbal sources are integrated by the episodic buffer. Information retrieved from long-term memory is processed in working memory before response in speech or action.

2) Deficits in working memory may affect the understanding of speech and written text. Finding the way in a known route and manipulating money for shopping may also be difficult. Competition for the limited resources in working memory for visual and verbal processing leads to difficulty in dual task performance.

3) The structure of long-term memory can be divided into declarative memory for facts and events that are explicitly retrieved, procedural or non-declarative memory for learnt motor and verbal skills which are implicit and without conscious access, and metamemory for prospective and evaluative aspects of memory. Prospective memory is a store of plans for future action and behaviour which usually have to be activated without external cues. Evaluative aspects include source monitoring and 'knowing what you know'.

4) Processing in long-term memory occurs in three stages. The first stage is registration at the time of learning, which depends on attention, the level of processing, elaboration and context. The second stage is retention over time, which is affected by modification and interference from new memories. The third stage is retrieval, which is achieved with or without awareness and is affected by context and mood.

5) Schema theory describes how stored knowledge relating to one situation (object, person, action or event) may be organised. Schemas develop because of experience and they guide top-down processing of incoming information to meet expectations.

6) The main brain areas involved in memory are the diencephalon, the medial temporal lobes and the frontal lobe. The hippocampus in the temporal lobe plays a pivotal role in the integration of memory systems. Long-term episodic and semantic memory can be selectively impaired, while procedural memory is usually spared. The features of amnesia include inability to learn new material, decay of stored memories and retrieval problems.

7) Long-term memory deficits result in loss of identity and independence. Social interaction with family and friends is severely affected by the loss of episodic memory. Participation in leisure games depends on memory aids for the semantic aspects such as scoring. Employment prospects are poor when the work involves a significant knowledge base. New learning is difficult and this becomes a hurdle in moving to a different job or home environment where novel ways of doing tasks must be learnt.

8) There are a range of standardised assessment tools for memory. Interventions tend to focus on compensatory strategies to aid function.

References

Ashcraft, M.H. and Radvansky, G.A. (2010) *Cognition*, 5th edn, Pearson/Prentice Hall, Upper Saddle River, New Jersey.

Baddeley, A. (2000) The episodic buffer: a new component of working memory? *Trends in Cognitive Science* (Regul. Ed.), **4** (11), 417–423.

Baddeley, A.D. (2007) *Working Memory, Thought and Action*, Oxford University Press, Oxford.

Baddeley, A.D. and Hitch, G.J. (1974) Working memory, in *Recent Advances in Learning and Motivation* (ed. G.A. Bower), Academic Press, New York, pp. 47–89.

Baddeley, A.D. and Wilson, B.A. (1988) Frontal amnesia and the dysexecutive syndrome. *Brain and Cognition*, **7** (2), 212–230.

Baddeley, A.D. and Wilson, B.A. (1994) When implicit learning fails: amnesia and the problem of error elimination. *Neuropsychologia*, **32**, 53–68.

Baddeley, A.D., Kopelman, M.D. and Wilson, B.A. (eds) (2002) *Handbook of Memory Disorders*, John Wiley, New York.

Baddeley, A.D., Eysenck, M.W. and Anderson, M.C. (2010) *Memory*, Psychology Press, New York.

Bartlett, F.C. (1932) *Remembering, A Study in Experimental and Social Psychology*, Cambridge University Press, New York.

Berry, J.M. and West, R.L. (1993) Cognitive self-efficacy in relation to personal mastery and goal setting across the life span. *International Journal of Behavioural Development*, **16** (2), 351–379.

Blaney, P.H. (1986) Affect and memory: a review. *Psychological Bulletin*, **99** (2), 229–246.

Brewer, W.F. and Treyens, J.C. (1981) Role of schemata in memory for places. *Cognitive Psychology*, **13**, 207–230.

Burke, J.M., Danick, J.A., Bemis, B. and Durkin, C.J. (1994) A process approach to memory book training for neurological patients. *Brain Injury*, **8** (1), 71–81.

Cicerone, K.D., Dahlberg, C., Malec, J.F. *et al.* (2005) Evidence-based cognitive rehabilitation: updated review of the literature from 1998–2002. *Archives of Physical Medicine and Rehabilitation*, **86**, 1681–1692.

Clare, L. and Jones, R. (2008) Errorless learning in the rehabilitation of memory impairment: a critical review. *Neuropsychological Review*, **18**, 1–23.

Cohen, G., Kiss, G. and LeVoi, M. (1993) *Memory: Current Issues*, Open University Press, Buckingham.

Conrad, R. (1964) Acoustic confusion in immediate memory. *British Journal of Psychology*, **55**, 75–84.

Conway, M. (2005) Memory and the self. *Journal of Memory and Language*, **53**, 594–628.

Conway, M., Pleydell-Pearce, C.W., Whitecross, S. and Sharpe, H. (2003) Neurophysiological correlates of memory for experienced and imagined events. *Neuropsychologia*, **41** (3), 334–340.

Craik, F.I.M. and Lockhart, R.S. (1972) Levels of processing. A framework for memory research. *Journal of Learning and Behaviour*, **11**, 671–684.

Craik, F.I.M. and Tulving, E. (1975) Depth of processing and the retention of words in episodic memory. *Journal of Experimental Psychology, General*, **104**, 268–294.

Cree, G.S. and McRae, K. (2003) Analysing the factors underlying the structure and computation of meaning of chipmunk, cherry, chisel, cheese and cello (and many other such concrete nouns). *Journal of Experimental Psychology, General*, **132**, 163–201.

Dalla Barba, G., Cipolotti, L. and Denes, G. (1990) Autobiographical memory loss and confabulation in Korsakoff's syndrome. *A case report. Cortex*, **26**, 525–534.

De Renzi, E., Liotti, M. and Nichelli, P. (1987) Semantic amnesia with preservation of autobiographical memory: a case report. *Cortex*, **23** (4), 575–597.

Fernandes, M.A. and Moscovitch, M. (2003) Interferences effects from divided attention during retrieval in younger and older adults. *Psychology of Ageing*, **18** (2), 219–230.

Fish, J., Manly, T., Emslie, H. and Evans, J.J. (2008) Compensatory strategies for acquired disorders of memory and planning: differential effects of a paging system for patients with brain injury of traumatic versus cerebrovascular aetiology. *Journal of Neurology, Neurosurgery, and Psychiatry*, **79** (8), 930–935.

Fish, J., Wilson, B.A. and Manly, T. (2010) The assessment and rehabilitation of prospective memory problems in people with neurological disorders. *Neuropsychological Rehabilitation*, **2**, 161–179.

Fleming, J.M., Shum, D., Strong, J. and Lightbody, S. (2005) Prospective memory rehabilitation for adults with traumatic brain injury: a compensatory training programme. *Brain Injury*, **19** (1), 1–10.

Folstein, M.F., Folstein, S.E. and McHugh, P.R. (1975) "Mini-mental state". A practical method for grading the cognitive state of patients for the clinician. *Journal of Psychiatric Research*, **12** (3), 189–198.

Glanzer, M. (1972) Mechanisms in recall, in *Recent Advances in Learning and Motivation* (ed. G.A. Bower), Academic Press, New York.

Greenberg, D.L. and Rubin, D.C. (2003) The neuropsychology of autobiographical memory. *Cortex*, **39** (4-5), 687–728.

Greenberg, D.L., Rice, H.J., Cooper, J.J. and Cabeze, R. (2005) Co-activation of the amygdala, hippocampus and inferior gyrus during autobiographical retrieval. *Neuropsychologia*, **43**, 659–674.

Hatano, G. and Osawa, K. (1983) Digit memory of grand experts in abacus-derived mental calculation. *Cognition*, **15**, 95–110.

Henry, J.D., MacLeod, M.S., Phillips, L.H. and Crawford, J.R. (2004) A meta-analytic review of prospective memory and ageing. *Psychology and Ageing*, **19**, 27–39.

Hildebrandt, H., Gehrmann, A., Modden, C. and Eling, P. (2011) Enhancing memory performance after organic brain disease relies on retrieval processes rather than encoding or consolidation. *Journal of Clinical and Experimental Neuropsychology*, **33** (2), 257–270.

Intercollegiate Stroke Working Party (2012) *National Clinical Guidelines for Stroke*, Royal College of Physicians, London.

Intercollegiate Stroke Working Party (2016) National Clinical Guidelines for Stroke, 5th edn., Available at: https://www.strokeaudit.org/Guideline/Full-Guideline.aspx (accessed 27th November 2016)

Jonides, J., Smith, E., Koeppe, R., Awh, E., Minoshima, S. and Mintum, M. (1993) Spatial working memory in humans as revealed by PET. *Nature*, **363**, 623–625.

Kalla, T., Downes, J.J. and de Broek, M. (2001) The pre-exposure technique: enhancing the effects of errorless learning in the association of face–name associations. *Neuropsychological Rehabilitation*, **11**, 1–16.

Levy, L.L. (2001) Memory processing and the older adult: what practitioners need to know. *Occupational Therapy Practice*, **6** (7), 1–8.

Maguire, E.A., Frackowiak, R.S.J. and Frith, C.D. (1997) Recalling routes around London: activation of the right hippocampus in taxi drivers. *Journal of Neuroscience*, **17**, 7103–7110.

Malia, K. and Brannagan, A. (2005) *How to Do Cognitive Rehabilitation Therapy: A Guide for All of Us*, Parts 1 and 2, Braintree Training, Leatherhead.

Meltzer, M.I. (1983) Poor memory: a case report. *Journal of Clinical Psychology*, **39** (1), 3–10.

Miller, G.A. (1956) The magical number seven, plus or minus two: some limits on our capacity for processing information. *Psychological Review*, **63**, 81–97.

Milner, B. (1966) Amnesia following operation on the temporal lobes, in *Amnesia* (eds C.W.M. Whitty and O.L. Zangwill), Butterworths, London, pp. 109–133.

Mioshi, E., Dawson, K., Mitchell, J., Arnold, R. and Hodges, J.R. (2006) The Addenbrooke's Cognitive Examination Revised (ACE-R): a brief cognitive test battery for dementia screening. *International Journal of Geriatric Psychiatry*, **21** (11), 1078–1085.

Morris, R. and Hannesdottir, K. (2004). Loss of 'awareness' in Alzheimer's disease, in *Cognitive Neuropsychology of Alzheimer's Disease* (eds R. Morris and J. Becker), Oxford University Press, Oxford.

Neisser, U. (1967) *Cognitive Psychology*, Appleton-Centaury Crofts, New York.

Page, M., Wilson, B.A., Shiel, A., Carter, G. and Norris, N. (2006).What is the locus of the errorless-learning advantage? *Neuropsychologia*, **44**, 90–100.

Parkinson, S.R., Inman, V.W. and Dannenbaum, S.E. (1985) Adult age differences in short term forgetting. *Acta Psychologica*, **60**, 83–101.

Pashler, H., Rohrer, D. and Cepeda, N.J. (2007) Enhancing learning and retarding forgetting: choices and consequences. *Psychonomic Bulletin and Review*, **14**, 187–193.

Paulesu, E., Frith, C.D. and Frackowiak, R.S.J. (1993) The neural correlates of the verbal component of working memory. *Nature*, **362**, 342–345.

Randolph, C., Tierney, M.C., Mohr, E. and Chase, T.N. (1998) The Repeatable Battery for the Assessment of Neuropsychological Status (RBANS): preliminary clinical validity. *Journal of Clinical and Experimental Neuropsychology*, **20** (3), 310–319.

Robbins, T.W., Anderson, E.J., Barker, D.R. and Bradley, A.C. (1996) Working memory in chess. *Memory and Cognition*, **24** (1), 83–93.

Royle, J. and Lincoln, N.B. (2008) The Everyday Memory Questionnaire-revised: development of a 13-item scale. *Disability and Rehabilitation*, **30** (2), 114–121.

Smith, G., del Sala, S., Logie, R.H. and Maylor, E.A. (2000) Prospective and respective memory in normal aging and dementia. *A questionnaire study. Memory*, **8**, 311–321.

Smith, R.E. and Bayen, U.J. (2005) The effects of working memory resource availability on prospective memory: a formal modelling approach. *Experimental Psychology*, **52**, 243–256.

Spiers, H.A., Maguire, E.A. and Burgess, N. (2001) Hippocampal amnesia. *Neurocase*, **7**, 357–382.

Squire, L.R. (1992) Declarative and non-declarative memory: multiple brain systems supporting learning and memory. *Journal of Cognitive Neuroscience*, **4**, 232–243.

Squire, L.R. (2009) Memory and brain systems: 1969–2009. *Journal of Neuroscience*, **29**, 12711–12716.

Sternberg, R.J. (1999) *Cognitive Psychology*, 2nd edn, Harcourt Brace College Publishers, Fort Worth, Texas.

Strayer, D.L. and Johnson, W.A. (2001) Driving to distraction: dual task studies of simulated driving and conversing on a cellular phone. *Psychological Science*, **12**, 462–466.

Sulin, R.A. and Dooling, D.J. (1974) Intrusion of a thematic idea in retention of prose. *Journal of Experimental Psychology*, **103**, 255–262.

Sunderland, A., Harris, J.D. and Baddeley, A.D. (1984) Assessing everyday memory after severe head injury, in *Everyday Memory, Actions and Absent Mindedness* (eds J.E. Harris and P. Morris), Academic Press, London.

Svoboda, E., McKinnon, M.C. and Levine, B. (2006) The functional neuroanatomy of autobiographical memory: a meta-analysis. *Neuropsychologia*, **44** (12), 2189–2208.

Thomson, J.A. (1983) Is continuous visual monitoring necessary in visually guided locomotion? *Journal of Experimental Psychology: Human Perception and Performance*, **9**, 427–443.

Tulving, E. (2002) Episodic memory: from mind to brain. *Annual Review of Psychology*, **53**, 1–25.

Tulving, E. & Thompson, D.M. (1973) Encoding specificity and retrieval processes in episodic memory. *Psychological Review*, **80** (5), 352–373.

Vogel, E.K., Woodman, J.F. and Luck, S.J. (2001) Storage of features, conjunctions and objects in visual working memory. *Journal of Experimental Psychology: Human Perception and Performance*, **27** (1), 92–114.

Warrington, E.K. and Weiskrantz, L. (1968) New methods of testing long term retention with special reference to amnesic patients. *Nature*, **217**, 972–974.

Wechsler, D. (2008) *Wechsler Adult Intelligence Scale*, 4th edn (WAIS–IV), NCS Pearson, San Antonio, Texas.

Weiskrantz, L. and Warrington, E.K. (1979) Conditioning in amnesic patients. *Neuropsychologia*, **8**, 281–288.

Wicklegrne, W.A. (1964) Size of rehearsal group and short term memory. *Journal of Experimental Psychology*, **68**, 413–419.

Williams, H.L., Conway, M.A. and Cohen, G. (2008) Autobiographical memory, in *Memory in the Real World*, 3rd edn (eds G. Cohen and M.A. Conway), Psychology Press, Hove, pp. 21–90.

Wilson, B.A. (2003) *Neuropsychological Rehabilitation: Theory and Practice (Studies on Neuropsychology, Development, and Cognition)*, Psychology Press, New York.

Wilson, B.A. and Wearing, D. (1995) Prisoner of consciousness: a state of just awakening following herpes simplex encephalitis, in *Broken Memories: Case Studies in Memory Impairment* (eds R. Campbell and M.A. Conway), Blackwell Publishing, Malden, Massachusetts, pp. 14–30.

Wilson, B.A., Emslie, H., Quirk, K. and Evans, J. (2005) A randomized control trial to evaluate a paging system for people with traumatic brain injury. *Brain Injury*, **19**, 891–894.

Wilson, B.A., Greenfield, E,. Clare, L. *et al.* (2008) *The Rivermead Behavioural Memory Test-3*, Pearson Assessment, London.

9

Purposeful Movement and Apraxia

Stephanie Tempest

AIMS
1) To outline the lived experience of apraxia.
2) To debate and clarify the terminology in the apraxia literature.
3) To explore the use of a neuropsychological model to aid our understanding of the praxis network.
4) To explore topics of gesture production and specific error types.
5) To consider assessment and intervention options.

Introduction

Cognition plays a major role in purposeful movements, all of which are goal directed. In order to carry out volitional activities, our cognitive skills need to interact with a range of performance skills, namely sensation and perception, memory and learning concepts, high-level executive functions, emotions and motor skills. The result of this interaction is the production of gestures; the two main ones we perform are those involving objects (tools) and those which are sociocultural, for example waving hello. These skills will be briefly explored in relation to gesture production, before focusing our attention on praxis and the absence of the ability to do purposeful movements, namely apraxia.

Cognition, Sensation and Perception

Sensory feedback about the position and movement of objects, or the interpretation of a sociocultural gesture, is incorporated into the planning of movement. For example, the manipulation of a glass includes tactile feedback about its weight, texture and fragility in order to determine the strength of grip required. We are aware of a mismatch between planning and perception if we pick up a carton of juice that is nearly empty when expecting it to be full or walk up an escalator that is not working. Sensory information (visual) is also required when interpreting facial expressions and body language.

Neuropsychology for Occupational Therapists: Cognition in Occupational Performance, Fourth Edition.
Edited by Linda Maskill and Stephanie Tempest.
© 2017 John Wiley & Sons Ltd. Published 2017 by John Wiley & Sons Ltd.
Companion Website: www.wiley.com/go/maskill/neuropsychologyOT

There is a significant sociocultural element here; for example, it may be harder to interpret hand gestures and tone of voice, as passionate or aggressive, if the person performing these gestures speaks a different language and is from a different culture to you.

Perceptual processing monitors the changing features of the environment during movement; errors are corrected based on the feedback from sensory input. Walking on different surfaces and around obstacles involves tactile input from the soles of the feet. The balance of the body is maintained by the integration of this cutaneous sensation with vision and proprioceptive information from the muscles and joints. Visuospatial perception allows us to orient the body in the correct position and direction, as we move around in space.

Cognition, Memory and Learning Concepts

Skilled activities and motor routines are developed with practice and stored in procedural memory. When the learned routine for riding a bicycle or driving a car is activated, the sequence of movements is performed automatically. During the progress along a route, declarative knowledge is retrieved into working memory for the recognition of landmarks recalled from occasions in the past. Remembering to act at some time in the future depends on prospective memory. The action may be triggered by a prompt, for example seeing a postbox when a letter needs to be posted, or we rely on our own strategy for initiating the action, for example holding the letter in our hand rather than putting it in a pocket out of sight.

High-Level Executive Functions

The executive functions enable us to deal with novel situations and challenges. Goals must be formulated and movements planned before initiation. The changing demands during the progress of an activity involve flexible problem solving to reach the goal, for example navigating a new route in the event that you are sent on a diversion and have left your satnav at home (or disagree with it!). Self-awareness and insight play a major role in purposeful activity to ensure we select the right response at the right time.

Emotion

Emotion has an effect on our attention to the task in hand and directly affects the quality of movement. In choosing how to act, incoming sensation and perceptual processing are integrated with our values and our emotional state at the time. Consider the example of a parent walking to collect their child from school. The mother may meet a neighbour who has been ill and wishes to chat. Emotional factors guide her decision whether to stop and talk or to be on time for her child at the end of the school day. There is evidence that the prefrontal area assesses the emotional quality of stimuli and influences decision making in movement.

The Production of Goal-Directed Purposeful Movement

Once sensory information has been processed and a variety of cognitive and psychosocial skills have interpreted the information, we are able to produce a goal-directed response. Elements within this final stage of purposeful movement include selecting the right response to generate the movement (involving memory) in order to organise a controlled response utilising our motor skills.

So, it is possible to see from this summary that task performance requires a complex interplay of many cognitive skills interacting with sensory, perceptual, emotional and motor skills. Indeed, the OTPF (AOTA 2014) acknowledges that performance skills encompass a multitude of motor, process and social interaction skills to enable a person to participate in activities and occupations.

Conceptualising and understanding the disorder of praxis skills, i.e. apraxia, has been described as a mystery by some. Indeed, the ICF (WHO 2001) does not use the term *praxis*, rather classifying 'the mental functions of sequencing complex movement' within the specific mental functions category. Therefore, in order to aid our understanding of the theory of praxis, first we will briefly outline the key terminologies within the praxis and apraxia literature.

Terminology in the Apraxia Literature

This section outlines some of the key terms common within the apraxia literature, namely imitation (concurrent and delayed), pantomime, gestures (transitive and intransitive), gesture identification and error types. In understanding these terms, we can begin to critically think about models of praxis and the underlying concepts which formulate our assessment tools. We will be exploring these concepts in more detail throughout this chapter.

Recent studies of praxis in neuropsychology have investigated the production of meaningful gestures. The results of these studies have shown that selective impairment of different types of gestures can occur. There are two main types of gesture production.

- *Imitation* – in this type, the person copies gestures that are made by the examiner, for example imitation of the movements for combing the hair. The imitation by the person may be done at the same time (concurrent imitation: CI) or after an interval of time (delayed imitation: DI).
- *Pantomime* – in this case, the person is asked to demonstrate a particular gesture, for example by responding to the command 'Show me how you would comb your hair'. In the case where a person also has communication difficulties, for example aphasia, they may be shown a picture of a hairbrush rather than a verbal instruction. The command is then followed by the person performing a mime of the action of hair combing. This type of gesture production demonstrates the ability of a person to generate a gesture from memory. The term *pantomime* relates to the original definition of the word as 'a show without words'.

Gestures performed by imitation (concurrent or delayed) and by pantomime may or may not involve objects. When an object is held in the hand, the gesture is tool based and known as *transitive*; for example, if the comb is held in the hand during pantomime, the gesture is transitive. Other gestures do not involve objects and are sociocultural by nature; these are known as *intransitive*. Examples are waving goodbye or the thumbs up sign.

Before a gesture is produced, the *gesture identification* process involves the brain possessing and utilising conceptual knowledge about how a gesture should be performed and the associated gesture linked to specific tools or actions. When there is a breakdown in the performance of gesture identification, imitation (concurrent or delayed) or pantomime – of transitive or intransitive gestures – error types are seen.

Error types are the product of an inability to perform goal-directed, purposeful gestures. Error types may comprise difficulties imitating and/or difficulties pantomiming specific tool or sociocultural gestures. Later in this chapter, we will explore some of the specific error types associated with apraxia and how they manifest in function.

When reading the literature on apraxia, whether it be in relation to understanding the nature of the impairment or for information on assessment and intervention, the terminology that has just been described is fundamental to aid our clinical reasoning. Therefore, it is essential that we feel comfortable in our understanding of imitation (concurrent and delayed), pantomime, gestures (transitive and intransitive), gesture identification and error types.

Models of Praxis

Praxis means movement and derives from the Greek for 'doing'. In this instance, it refers to the doing of volitional, goal-directed and purposeful movement. As we have discussed, praxis is a complex interplay between motor, sensory, perceptual, psychosocial and cognitive processes. Yet apraxia is commonly considered a cognitive impairment, the definition of which will be explored later. This is not a new concept as, in the nineteenth century, neurologists were describing non-motor components involved in the production of movement:

> 'There is power in his muscles and in the centres for co-ordination of muscular groups, but he, the whole man or the "will", cannot set them agoing.'
> *(Hughlings Jackson 1866, cited in Brown 1988)*

Our understanding of the production of purposeful movement is enhanced through the exploration of models of praxis. There are two main ways to view apraxia: neuroanatomical correlates seeking to locate the parts of the brain responsible for praxis and neuropsychological models identifying the systems and levels of processing involved.

Neuroanatomical Correlates

In 1905, the neurologist Hugo Liepmann was one of the first people to identify a specific motor planning and praxis network within the brain. He postulated the role of the left hemisphere, especially the left parietal lobe, as dominant for purposeful movement as well as language. The left parietal lobe projects to the left frontal motor areas for movements of the right (dominant) side of the body and via the corpus callosum for the left (non-dominant) side. The early neuroanatomical model of praxis outlined a system for integration of:

- the left parietal lobe which stores semantic (conceptual) knowledge of objects and action plans related to their use with
- the motor areas in the frontal lobes which execute the correct spatial and temporal features of gestures and object-oriented movements.

As our understanding has developed, the critique of the early neuroanatomical model of praxis is that it is oversimplified, as there is a need to distinguish between different sensory inputs and also to explain the role of stored motor programmes.

Nonetheless, it was Liepmann who first highlighted a movement disorder associated with the use of tools and objects. He also distinguished between the idea and the execution/motor aspect of purposeful movement, although some have debated whether this distinction has led to continued confusion regarding distinct types of apraxia (Hanna-Pladdy and Gonzales Rothi 2001).

Neuroimaging studies continue to support the role of the parietal and frontal lobes in the left hemisphere within praxis, but there is evidence to suggest the involvement of the right hemisphere (Haaland *et al.* 2000), occipital and temporal lobes (Makuuchi *et al.* 2005) and subcortical locations (Pramstaller and Marsden 1996). These studies support the notion that there is a widespread neural praxis network within the brain and the ability to perform meaningful movements is not exclusive to the left parietal lobe.

Neuropsychological Models

Rather than focusing on identifying specific parts of the brain responsible for praxis, cognitive neuropsychology seeks to conceptualise, through models, the processes involved with producing goal-directed movements but the debates continue to this day, and have done so for at least the last century.

One model of the stages of processing was initially developed by Roy and Square (1994, as outlined in Roy 1996) and was updated by Stamenova *et al.* (2012). This updated version of the conceptual-production systems model was validated using data from 73 people with stroke and 27 healthy matched subjects and is shown in Figure 9.1.

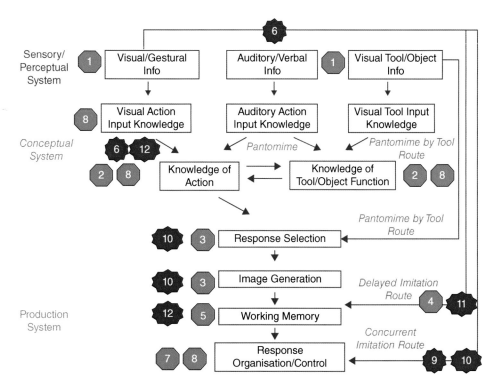

Figure 9.1 Conceptual-production systems model. The numerals denote different apraxic performance patterns identified by the research team as detailed in the article. Source: Stamenova *et al.* (2012). Reproduced with permission of Elsevier.

Three stages of processing are described, but these are not in a hierarchy and stages can be by-passed.

- *Sensory/perceptual system* which makes a distinction between visual, auditory and object information demonstrated by performance in different types of gesture.
- *Conceptual system* which is the semantic system for knowledge of object function and the movements related to their use. The output from the first level accesses this stored knowledge of actions associated with objects and with sociocultural gestures, for example waving goodbye.
- *Production system* which organises and controls response selection and generates the correct innervatory patterns for the movements.

In the model shown in Figure 9.1, the numbers 1–12 indicate different gestural/apraxic deficit patterns. So, for example, pattern 6 is *P+/DI-/CI-/ID+* and this translates as pantomime skills intact; delayed imitation impaired; concurrent imitation impaired; gesture identification intact.

Activity
Write in full the presentation of pattern 7 = P-/DI-/CI-/ID+

Our understanding of the terminology in the apraxia literature is central to appreciating the conceptual-production model of limb apraxia. Imitation of gestures is divided into concurrent imitation (CI) and delayed imitation (DI) which rely on different memory structures.

The CI route (see Figure 9.1) involves a person performing a gesture (either transitive or intransitive) concurrently with the examiner; for example, both mime the act of hair combing at the same time. In this case, visual gestural information directly accesses the response organisation and control stage.

The DI route is used when the person relies on someone else performing the intransitive or transitive gesture; for example, an examiner mimes combing the hair and the person copies the gesture later. In using the DI route, the person needs to store the movements in working memory before imitation on completion of the demonstration. A person who is unable to pantomime a gesture from long-term memory may be able to perform delayed imitation of gestures via working memory.

A person who is able to do imitation is demonstrating that they are still able to process visual/gestural information. Concurrent imitation is the only possible route for someone with impaired working memory.

Returning to the model shown in Figure 9.1, the early stages of processing are associated with analysing in parallel: visual gestural information; auditory input from commands; and visual tool/object input. The next stage involves integration with semantic processing of knowledge of object function and the actions associated with their use. The later stages include response selection and/or image generation which translates the conceptual knowledge into action. The final stage is the organisation and control of the response which includes movement sequencing and co-ordination.

Understanding Apraxia

Living with Apraxia

In the description below (adapted from Blijlevens *et al.* 2009 and Arntzen and Elstad 2013), it is evident that life with apraxia means that the smallest tasks can take a lot of time or can be impossible to do. Sometimes a person knows they are using the wrong tool but are unable to do anything about it. The support and attitudes of those around the person are crucial in adapting to life with apraxia.

People with apraxia make errors when performing activities using objects and tools or when performing sociocultural gestures. Errors are reduced in a familiar environment, for example brushing the teeth in the bathroom at home, because such environments provide cues that prompt well-learned movement sequences.

Single actions, such as putting a plug into a socket or turning on the tap, may be done fluently but the situation changes when an activity involves sequencing a series of actions and the use of more than one object. The component actions in a sequence may be in the wrong order, or a stage is omitted, for example stirring a coffee mug with no water in it, or two parts of the sequence may be blended together. Sequencing in dressing is usually unique to the individual. Some people dress the lower body before the

---

The lived experience of apraxia

You've got to be prepared to devote time to doing the smallest of things. Getting dressed takes the best part of half an hour; the biggest problem for me is buttons as they just keep sliding away all the time. It is like my hand takes its own way. I can't hang clothes on the line and that makes me feel pretty small and frustrated. Sometimes I know what I'm doing is wrong, so the other day I tried to cut a slice of bread with a table knife, but I couldn't do anything about it. And other days, I blame the things around me and say things like 'The coffee maker was stupid today... perhaps as stupid as me'.

But there is stuff that healthcare professionals and those around us can do to help; because how I feel can depend on the staff and their attitude – if they don't know what they are doing, it's quite degrading. So I tell them not to rush me, or I lose my memory of how to put my jacket on; I ask them to give me time and space to help me be competent at something and I remind them to support hopefulness that things will improve. It helps if they try to understand what I am experiencing.

I've also found it enormous help to talk to other people with apraxia, it helps us all to adapt, recover and develop our own language to discuss our experiences. Healthcare professionals could learn from us to increase their own knowledge of the strategies we have discovered that help us do our daily activities.

Activity

Write down the key messages that you have heard from those living with apraxia to inform your own therapeutic approach.

upper body and vice versa. In apraxia, sequencing errors may lead to underclothes being donned on top of trousers.

Some people with apraxia can perform object-based activities but struggle with sociocultural gestures. A hand offered in greeting may not result in the person grasping and shaking it. This may be due to the inability to recognise the gesture (conceptual error) or the person is unable to produce the movement in response (production error). It is possible to see how this could be misinterpreted by someone unfamiliar with the impact of the impairment who subsequently may erroneously conclude that the person with apraxia is being rude.

Some people with apraxia are unaware of the errors they are making and are in danger of causing accidents, such as leaving the gas unlit on the cooker. In other instances, the person is aware of the errors being made but can do nothing to correct them. They may be wrongly labelled as confused.

In the familiar home environment, there may be no problems with routine and habitual tasks that can be completed automatically. When the attentional demands increase, the movements lack fluency and look clumsy. This can be a source of irritation to the individual and the family. In the absence of other problems, the person with apraxia can function reasonably well at home but safety may always remain a concern.

Definitions of Apraxia

The most cited definition of apraxia is from Geschwind (1975) who described the apraxias as disorders of the execution of learned movement in the absence of weakness, inco-ordination, sensory loss, incomprehension or inattention to commands. However, there are difficulties with this definition as it is based on exclusion criteria and therefore defines what apraxia is not.

Apraxia has also been defined as a disorder affecting the ability to pantomime or imitate gestures (Roy and Square 1994), which helps to qualify the impact of the impairment, and also as a disorder of higher motor cognition (Dovern *et al.* 2012), which helps to quantify its complex and multifaceted nature.

Within occupational therapy, there is sometimes additional confusion as the terms *dyspraxia* and *apraxia* have been used interchangeably. Ayres (1985) reported that there is a distinction to make between apraxia and dyspraxia, stating that apraxia is a disorder of learned movement and therefore occurs in adults with acquired neurological disorders; the praxis ability was once present and now it is absent (hence the prefix 'a'). This tends to be a disorder affecting the conceptual or production stages of volitional movement as described in the conceptual production system model previously. In contrast, dyspraxia is a disorder of new learning of motor patterns and sequences, therefore potentially referring to children who have difficulties acquiring praxis skills (hence the prefix 'dys'). Dyspraxia is often viewed as a disorder affecting the sensory stage of volitional movement, hence the development of sensory integration techniques when working with children. However, there is also debate within the paediatric field concerning the use of the term *dyspraxia* at all, with some diagnostic manuals and guidelines using the term developmental co-ordination disorder (DCD).

The neuropsychological literature consistently uses the term *apraxia* when discussing impairment of volitional movement in adults with acquired brain injury. The distinction goes beyond semantics. If a person has previously learned motor patterns and praxis ability, this may be harnessed within their rehabilitation, for example using mental imagery to recall how to ride a bicycle. On the other hand, the focus of intervention for children with developmental difficulties may need to enhance new learning, for example, if they have not yet learnt to ride a bicycle.

'Different Types' of Apraxia Versus Different Gestural Deficit Patterns

Geschwind (1975) referred to multiple apraxias and indeed, there are over 30 different types recorded in the literature including buccofacial, constructional, dressing, gait, gaze, limb and speech apraxia. The term *apraxia* is applied to each of these disorders, many of which are unrelated in their origin. Dressing apraxia has been challenged as a distinct type because it could be argued that the difficulty in dressing is the functional manifestation of the impairment or is caused by a number of impairments.

The two most common types of apraxia, *ideational* and *ideomotor*, will first be described before we debate the usefulness of labelling 'different types' and propose an alternative for consideration.

Ideational apraxia has been described as an 'agnosia of usage' which is loss of the knowledge of the use of objects. This definition can be mapped on to the conceptual-production systems model (Stamenova *et al.* 2012) at the level of the conceptual system (see Figure 9.1). Therefore, ideational apraxia is understood as a disorder in the performance of purposeful movement due to a loss of the conceptual (semantic) knowledge of movement related to objects. This loss of action memories associated with object function means that visual and auditory information, related to the function of objects, cannot access the conceptual system and the pantomime of gestures is impaired. Imitation remains intact as the visual/gestural route can still be utilised (see Figure 9.1).

Errors are made when using objects and tools in routine task performance and on command. People with ideational apraxia may be able to name and describe the function of objects using visual and tactile information, but they cannot integrate this knowledge with the actions related to their use due to the breakdown at the conceptual level of motor performance.

Ideomotor apraxia is defined as a disorder in the selection, timing and spatial organisation of purposeful movement causing difficulties in making an organised and controlled motor response. This is a disruption to the production system as defined by Stamenova *et al.* (2012) (see Figure 9.1). A person with ideomotor apraxia cannot carry out what is intended and has impaired imitation and/or pantomime. This differs from ideational apraxia where imitation is intact. Errors are made when the person is asked to perform object-oriented movements both on verbal command (pantomime) and by copying the examiner (imitation). The spatial and temporal features of the movements are most affected.

There is a debate within the literature about whether ideational and ideomotor apraxia are distinct impairments. As previously mentioned, the persisting confusion has been related back to the original work by Liepmann because he was the first to make a distinction between the idea and the execution. However, using the conceptual-production system model (Stamenova *et al.* 2012), it is evident that apraxia is caused by breakdowns at several different levels which are all part of the same praxis network. Ideational apraxia relates to breakdown at the conceptual level and ideomotor apraxia refers to the production stage. So it could be argued that ideational and ideomotor apraxia are overlapping disorders that lie on the same continuum.

As occupational therapists working with people who have difficulties producing goal-directed movement, it may be better to focus on and describe the different gestural deficit patterns with which a person with apraxia presents, for example P-/DI-/CI-/ID+, leaving clinicians to classify the type of apraxia in their favoured classification scheme (Dovern *et al.* 2012). So, rather than seeking to label someone as having a specific type of apraxia, it could be more clinically useful and more meaningful to the person with apraxia to identify, in function, if they can imitate (concurrent and/or delayed), pantomime, identify gestures and the error types that present. The latter will now be explored in more detail. Indeed, analysis of functional performance is firmly rooted in our professional domain whereas prescribing diagnostic labels is not.

Error Types in Performance

Different error types that are observed within function enable occupational therapists to distinguish apraxia-related impairments from other motor impairments, for example hemiplegia. The error types that are produced depend on the level at which the breakdown in performance occurs, i.e. sensory, conceptual or production. It must be appreciated that the error types observed in function tend to be at the conceptual or production stages because they are the tangible aspects of volitional movement.

Research continues to identify different apraxic error types. Table 9.1 lists some of the error types that have been identified to date together with functional examples associated with each.

Table 9.1 Common error types and functional manifestations for a person with apraxia.

Error type	Functional example
Omission	A step within a task is left out, e.g. does not put paste on the toothbrush
Difficulty terminating movements (NB: different from perseveration – see below)	Continues to stir the coffee for a prolonged period
Repetitions (NB: also different from perseveration)	Washing the same body part again
Disturbances to order of movements in sequence	Attempts to pour the milk from the bottle without removing the lid
Difficulties co-ordinating limbs in time and space	May overshoot when reaching for the kettle or have difficulty with tasks that require the use of both upper limbs
Perseveration	Performs the same movement in two consecutive activities, e.g. stirs the coffee then stirs the sugar instead of spooning action
Performance in wrong plane	May wave goodbye with a flat hand
Using body part as object	Using hand to comb hair
Verbalise performance without completing	Able to talk through the steps required but not able to complete the actions
Poor performance to verbal command, e.g. 'Show me how you would butter the toast'	Presses the butter into the toast with a knife instead of spreading it
Mismatching object to action	Attempts to comb hair with a tube of sweets

There is no definitive number of error types required for a person to be identified as having apraxia. It should be noted that errors may be compounded by other factors, such as the role of the environment. Some people can function within their home environment but may make errors when asked to perform the same activities in an unfamiliar one, for example wash and dress by the hospital bed. Moreover, some people are able to use objects and tools whilst struggling with sociocultural gestures such as waving goodbye to a relative. This warrants the recommendation to use a standardised assessment to identify apraxia in conjunction with a functional one (Intercollegiate Stroke Working Party 2016).

In the last 40 years, over 20 tests have been devised for apraxia and these often measure different components within the impairment (Dovern *et al.* 2012). Current clinical guidelines for stroke in England and Wales (Intercollegiate Stroke Working Party 2016) recommend the use of a standardised tool, for example the Test of Upper Limb Apraxia (TULIA) (Vanbellingen *et al.* 2010). The TULIA measures a person's ability to imitate and pantomime but it does not measure actual object use so it needs to be used as part of an overall assessment package including functional assessment.

Butler (2002) argued that it may be more clinically relevant for occupational therapists to consider functional and behavioural indices in activities of daily living rather than strive for test scores within the assessment process. Functional assessments for apraxia have been identified in the literature (e.g. Goldenberg and Hagmann 1998) and other assessment tools, for example the Assessment of Motor and Process Skills (AMPS) (Fisher 1999), identify underlying skills within a given functional situation. This adds further weight to the argument that when working with people who present with apraxia, it is more important to focus on the gestural abilities and functional consequences of the impairment rather than spending time identifying the 'type' of apraxia.

Activity

Mr MFP, aged 72, is a film producer who had an extensive middle cerebral artery infarct. On admission to the rehabilitation unit, he did not have independent sitting balance and he had no functional use of his right arm. He was unable to speak or understand verbal instruction. Standardised tests were inappropriate and observation of function was used. When attempting to eat slices of banana, he would overshoot when reaching for them. He occasionally took his hand to his mouth without a piece of banana present, or when present he would bring the food to his mouth with his wrist in flexion and hand in pronation.

Using the information from this case study, discuss how you might identify the level(s) where the breakdown in performance occurs for MFP, using the conceptual-production model of Stamenova *et al.* (2012).

Suggestions for Assessment and Intervention

Assessment

- Use activities that require both transitive (tool-based) and intransitive (sociocultural) gestures.
- Ascertain if a person is able to pantomime and imitate (both concurrent and delayed). Ask them to perform an activity to verbal command with and without the

object present, and then use a photograph as a cue (also helpful if communication skills are impaired). Relate this information to the conceptual-production model of praxis to determine the level(s) of breakdown in performance and the pattern of gestural deficit.

- Observe function within a naturalistic environment whenever possible.
- Document the types of errors observed and note if the person is able to overcome them (reparable) or if the errors are fatal (i.e. the therapist needs to intervene to aid continuation of the task).
- Consider the different stages of goal-directed movement and observe at which stage the breakdown may be occurring: sensory/perceptual, conceptual or production stages.

Assessment Resources

As mentioned, the TULIA (Vanbellingen *et al.* 2010) is recommended and a short screening version has also been devised (Vanbellingen *et al.* 2011). Other standardised assessment tools measure apraxia within the component sections and these include the LOTCA and the AMPS.

Intervention

- Provide and/or teach compensatory strategies (Intercollegiate Stroke Working Party 2016).
- Explain the impairment and the impact on function to the person, their family and their treating team (Intercollegiate Stroke Working Party 2016).
- Be careful if thinking about issuing equipment (new tools, for example a bathboard), as a new transitive gesture for someone with difficulties performing existing transitive gestures could prove too difficult. You may need to introduce essential equipment through a process of chaining.
- *Strategy training* – teach the person and their family the concept of activity analysis and chaining; they may wish to transfer this technique to other priority activities and take control of their own rehabilitation.
- Carry out intervention sessions within the naturalistic environment wherever possible and use items within the environment for non-verbal cues.
- Intervention must be task specific and the activity must be a meaningful priority for the client.
- As appropriate, use hand over hand guidance, imitation (delayed or concurrent) and/or pantomime techniques. So, as the therapist, you may wish to perform the gesture first – to be copied after – or do the movement at the same time.
- Use an errorless learning approach and repetition, intervening before errors occur to facilitate learning and improve function.
- Minimise the amount of verbal cues – there is a high association between apraxia and communication difficulties.
- Aim to improve function despite the persistence of apraxia and not 'cure' the impairment, i.e. compensation.
- Understand that you are intervening to manage the impairment rather than treat it (aiming for adaptation of performance or compensation, rather than remediation).

Sources of Evidence for Interventions

- Activity analysis, chaining (Wilson 1988)
- Combined mental and physical practice (Wu *et al.* 2011)
- Gesture training (Smania *et al.* 2000, 2006)
- Direct training (Goldenberg *et al.* 2001)
- Strategy training (Geusgens *et al.* 2006)

SUMMARY

1) The ability to perform goal-directed activities involves a complex network of sensory, perceptual, emotional, cognitive and motor skills. Studies of neuroanatomical correlates associated with apraxia identify a number of neural sites, both cortical and subcortical, although the left parietal lobe plays a dominant role.

2) The conceptual-production system model of limb praxis developed by Roy and Square (1996) and subsequently validated and revised by Stamenova *et al.* (2012) identifies three stages to produce purposeful movement: sensory/perceptual, conceptual (semantic) and production systems. Apraxia is a higher motor cognitive disorder that affects the ability to generate the idea of a movement and/or execute a purposeful movement. Ideational and ideomotor apraxia are different but interrelated types of apraxia caused by breakdown at different levels within the praxis network.

3) Understanding the terminology within the apraxia literature is crucial to aid our clinical reasoning for assessment and intervention strategies. The therapist needs to assess if a person is able to pantomime gestures (i.e. perform from memory), to imitate (concurrently and in a delayed manner) and identify gestures. There are two main types of gestures: transitive (tool based) and intransitive (sociocultural). Error types, of which a number of specific types are defined in the literature, can occur in both types of gesture production.

4) Assessment of apraxia should focus on gesture production and functional performance rather than attempting to define a specific type.

5) Intervention should seek to improve function despite the persistence of the impairment. Working with the person with apraxia, and those close to them, is crucial in raising awareness about the impairment and how it can be overcome. Healthcare professionals can also learn much from people with apraxia in terms of compensatory strategies and how to support hopefulness.

References

American Occupational Therapy Association (2014) Occupational therapy practice framework: Domain and process, 3rd ed. *American Journal of Occupational Therapy,* **68** (Suppl. 1), S1–S48.

Arntzen, C. and Elstad, I. (2013) The bodily experience of apraxia in everyday activities: a phenomenological study. *Disability and Rehabilitation,* **35** (1), 63–72.

Ayres, A.J. (1985) *Developmental dyspraxia and adult-onset apraxia.* A lecture prepared for Sensory Integration International, Torrance, California.

Blijlevens, H., Hocking, C. and Paddy, A. (2009) Rehabilitation of adults with dyspraxia: health professionals learning from patients. *Disability and Rehabilitation*, **31** (6), 466–475.

Brown, J. (1988) *Agnosia and Apraxia: Selected Papers of Liepmann, Lange and Potzl*, Lawrence Erlbaum, Hillsdale, New Jersey.

Butler, J. (2002) How comparable are tests of apraxia? *Clinical Rehabilitation*, **16** (4), 389–398.

Dovern, A., Fink, G.R. and Weiss, P.H. (2012) Diagnosis and treatment of upper limb apraxia. *Journal of Neurology*, **259**, 1269–1283.

Fisher, A. (1999) *The Assessment of Motor and Process Skills*, 3rd edn, Three Star, Fort Collins, Colorado.

Geschwind, N. (1975) The apraxias: neural mechanisims of disorders of learned movement. *American Scientist*, **63**, 188–195.

Geusgens, C., van Heugten, C., Donkervoort, M., van den Ende, E., Jolles, J. and van den Heuvel, W. (2006) Transfer of training effects in stroke patients with apraxia: an exploratory study. *Neuropsychological Rehabilitation*, **16** (2), 213–229.

Goldenberg, G. and Hagmann, S. (1998) Therapy of activities of daily living in patients with apraxia. *Neuropsychological Rehabilitation*, **8** (2), 123–141.

Goldenberg, G., Daumuller, M. and Hagmann, S. (2001) Assessment and therapy of complex activities of daily living in apraxia. *Neuropsychological Rehabilitation*, **11** (2), 147–169.

Haaland, K., Harrington, D. and Knight, R. (2000) Neural representations of skilled movement. *Brain*, **123** (11), 2306–2313.

Hanna-Pladdy, B. and Gonzales Rothi, L.J. (2001) Ideational apraxia: confusion that began with Liepmann. *Neuropsychological Rehabilitation*, **11** (5), 539–547.

Intercollegiate Stroke Working Party (2016) *National Clinical Guidelines for Stroke*, 5th edn. Available at: https://www.strokeaudit.org/Guideline/Full-Guideline.aspx (accessed 27th November 2016).

Makuuchi, M., Kaminaga, T. and Sugishita, M. (2005) Brain activation during ideomotor praxis: imitation and movements executed by verbal command. *Journal of Neurology, Neurosurgery and Psychiatry*, **76**, 25–33.

Pramstaller, P. and Mardsen, C.D. (1996) The basal ganglia and apraxia. *Brain*, **119**, 319–340.

Roy, E.A. (1996) Hand preference, manual asymmetries and limb apraxia, in *Manual Asymmetries in Motor Control* (eds D. Elliott and E.A. Roy), CRC Press, Boca Raton, Florida.

Roy, E.A. and Square, P.A. (1994) Neuropsychology of movement sequencing disorders and apraxia, in *Neuropsychology* (ed. D.W. Zaidel), Academic Press, San Diego, California, pp. 185–214.

Smania, N., Girardi, F., Domenicali, C., Lora, E. and Aglioti, S. (2000) The rehabilitation of limb apraxia: a study in left-brain damaged patients. *Archives of Physical Medicine and Rehabilitation*, **81**, 379–388.

Smania, N., Aglioti, S.M., Firardi, F. *et al.* (2006) Rehabilitation of limb apraxia improves daily life activities in patients with stroke. *Neurology*, **67**, 2050–2052.

Stamenova, V., Black, S. and Roy, E.A. (2012) An update on the conceptual-production systems model of limb apraxia: evidence from stroke. *Brain and Cognition*, **80**, 53–63.

Vanbellingen, T., Kersten, B., van Hemelrijk, B. *et al.* (2010) Comprehensive assessment of gesture production: a new test of upper limb apraxia (TULIA). *European Journal of Neurology*, **17**, 59–66.

Vanbellingen, T., Kersten, B., van de Winckel, A. *et al.* (2011) A new bedside test of gestures in stroke: the apraxia screen of TULIA (AST). *Journal of Neurology, Neurosurgery and Psychiatry*, **82**, 389–392.

Wilson, B.A. (1988) Sarah: remediation of apraxia following an anaesthetic accident, in *Clinical Psychology in Action: A Collection of Case Studies* (eds J. West and P. Spinks), Butterworth, London.

World Health Organisation (2001) *International Classification of Functioning, Disability and Health (ICF)*, World Health Organisation, Geneva.

Wu, A.J., Radel, J. and Hanna-Pladdy, B. (2011) Improved function after combined physical and mental practice after stroke: a case of hemiparesis and apraxia. *American Journal of Occupational Therapy*, **65**, 161–168.

10

Executive Functions

Sacha Hildebrandt

AIMS

1) To outline the lived experience of executive dysfunction.
2) To describe the higher-level cognitive skills comprised within executive functioning.
3) To explore neuroanatomical and neuropsychological explanations to aid our understanding of executive dysfunction.
4) To consider assessment and intervention options.

What are Executive Functions?

The term *executive function* or *executive functioning* can be a source of considerable confusion. Executive functions do not represent a unitary cognitive concept but rather the co-ordinated combination of a host of cognitive processes that allow an individual to function at the highest level at home, at school and at work. We might think of executive functions as fulfilling the role of a chairperson or chief executive of a large corporation. They are responsible for integrating and co-ordinating all the employees and component parts of the business to ensure its successful and effective operation.

Executive functioning is considered the highest level of cognitive function; its efficiency and effectiveness depend on the dynamic and 'online' integration and co-ordination of other cognitive functions including orientation, memory, attention, insight and awareness.

From the moment we wake up until we go to sleep again at night, human beings operate within a range of changing environments that influence and affect our behaviour and vice versa. Many activities are routine, such as brushing our teeth or showering, and require very little online attention and focus to complete. Others are novel and demand the ability to process information quickly, to make a judgement as to how best to respond (considering all factors involved), to plan and execute an appropriate response, to monitor the quality of our actions and adjust these accordingly, and finally to complete the job

Neuropsychology for Occupational Therapists: Cognition in Occupational Performance, Fourth Edition.
Edited by Linda Maskill and Stephanie Tempest.
© 2017 John Wiley & Sons Ltd. Published 2017 by John Wiley & Sons Ltd.
Companion Website: www.wiley.com/go/maskill/neuropsychologyOT

at hand. This can be something minor, such as finding out that you have run out of milk so you are unable to have your usual cereal for breakfast, or more complicated, for example, roadworks on your drive to work that prevent you from taking your usual route. To address both of these situations, we require intact executive functions.

A single definition of executive functioning remains elusive although common components within definitions include the notion that they are required in complex, sometimes novel, problem-solving situations, when behaviour must be modified in light of new information (Elliott 2003). Within this band of higher level cognitive skills are abstract thinking, the ability to organise and plan, time management, cognitive flexibility, insight, judgement and problem solving (WHO 2001).

Executive functions have been broadly divided into 'cold' and 'hot' components. The skills previously outlined refer to the 'cold' cognitive components which are relatively mechanistic and logically based (Chen *et al.* 2008). However, there is little reference made to the 'hot' components which are also deemed to be an important part of executive functioning. These involve emotions, beliefs and desires, and include interpersonal skills, social behaviour, personality and interpreting complex emotions (Chen *et al.* 2008; Damasio 1994). The ICF considers these skills as global mental functions or personal factors (WHO 2001) so there are differences in how they are classified. However, the key point to be appreciated is that when considering executive functioning, we must remember that there is a complex interplay between the 'hot' and 'cold' components.

Categories of Executive Functions

Broadly speaking, executive functions can be divided into the following categories, all of which encompass hot and cold components when applied to everyday life.

- Initiation and inhibition
- Goal setting/intentionality
- Planning and organisation
- Self-monitoring and problem solving

To be effective, these categories are reliant on a degree of insight and self-awareness and intact underlying attention and working memory systems. They will be individually explored in the following subsections.

Initiation and Inhibition

It is known that the executive system is involved in initiating action, either self-generated through an internal drive to act or in response to an environmental cue. The latter is easier as it is prompted, such as being asked a question, whereas self-generating an action, for example striking up conversation or getting up in the morning to get ready for work, is more cognitively challenging (Bell 2006).

Of equal importance are the following performance skills: terminating a response and inhibiting an automatic or habitual response. Disinhibition and impulsivity are the behavioural consequences of problems with these skills (Burgess *et al.* 1998), for example not being able to walk past a closed door without trying to open it or not being able to stop yourself making an inappropriate comment about a passer-by's unusual outfit.

Goal Setting/Intentionality

Goal-related behaviour requires an individual to create, activate and maintain a purposeful plan of action (Burgess *et al.* 1998). Goals and subgoals are crucial in governing human behaviour in response to environmental and internal demands (Levine *et al.* 2000). One of the main purposes of having goals is to impose structure on behaviour by controlling the initiation or inhibition of actions that either facilitate or prevent task completion. The frontal lobe is involved in goal-directed and goal-oriented action, and when there is damage, an individual may be unable to identify appropriate goals. If they are able to remember intended goals, they are unable to execute them in an organised and timely manner or to achieve completion. This has been referred to as goal neglect (Chen *et al.* 2008). Interestingly, insight and awareness, mediated largely by the right frontal lobe, are closely linked to goal setting and intentionality. It is argued that only if we have an accurate awareness of our abilities and our social and physical environment are we able to accurately, appropriately and realistically direct our behaviour accordingly (Stuss and Alexander 2000).

Planning and Organisation

Being able to identify an appropriate goal is challenging for some individuals, but being able to plan how, when, with what or with whom you will implement and execute the multiple actions of the goal to its completion is much more demanding. Functions of attention and working memory are thought to play a pivotal role in these planning and organisational processes. These skills enable individuals to remain focused in the presence of distraction, and to keep track of where they are in the process of goal completion. Many people with brain injuries show an overall 'life disorganisation' with a poor ability to manage and attain goals even if they are able to explain their intentions at the outset, as they present with distractibility and poor retention of information (Novakovic-Agopian *et al.* 2011).

Self-Monitoring and Problem Solving

Self-monitoring and problem solving require us to review our behaviour, in response to the environment, and chart our progress in pursuing goals. We also need to constantly assess whether our behaviour and efforts are too much, too little, appropriate, inappropriate, on track or going awry. It is also the ability to recognise when a selected action has failed or errors have occurred, and to be able to select a different strategy or adapt our behaviour to solve the problem and ensure goal attainment. Being adaptable and flexible in response to changing circumstances is essential for effective goal completion and everyday function (Levine *et al.* 2000), and is also reliant on having good insight and awareness.

Neuroanatomy

Historically, 'executive functions' and 'frontal lobe function' were terms used interchangeably as it was believed that only people with frontal lobe damage, caused most commonly by traumatic brain injury, would present with the above-mentioned difficulties. Neuroimaging studies showed that the prefrontal cortex within the frontal lobes was clearly implicated as a key determinant of executive function. However, more recent research indicates that this is too simplistic; first, this is a heterogenous region and therefore different areas of the prefrontal cortex are responsible for different executive functions. Second, subcortical regions and corticostriatal circuitry can also be involved (Elliott 2003).

With reference to the 'cold' and 'hot' components of executive functions, it is believed that the dorsolateral area of the prefrontal cortex is broadly responsible for the former whilst the orbitofrontal or ventromedial area is broadly responsible for the latter (Chen *et al.* 2008).

Causes of Executive Dysfunction

Traumatic brain injury (TBI), through its effects upon the ascending systems involved in arousal and regulation, and the ventral frontal and anterior temporal cortices, is among the most common causes of executive dysfunction (Levine *et al.* 2000). It has been found that numerous diagnoses other than TBI share similar impairments. These include Huntington's disease, multiple systems atrophy, progressive supranuclear palsy and Parkinson's disease (Elliot 2003). People with psychiatric disorders such as schizophrenia and depression suffer from executive dysfunction, as do people with Alzheimer's and AIDS-related dementia (Elliot 2003). It has also been reported that as many as 75% of stroke survivors experience some degree of executive dysfunction (Chung *et al.* 2013), and that natural ageing may negatively affect executive functions as the prefrontal cortex shows signs of atrophy (Andres and van der Linden 2000).

Models of Executive Function

The following models, all devised through analysis of the adult population, may help to further clarify the nature of executive functions.

Luria's Theory

Luria (1966) proposed that the human brain comprised three functional units that were interactively linked. The first unit is based in the brainstem and regulates arousal of the cortex. The second unit is based in the temporal, parietal and occipital lobes and is responsible for processing, encoding and storing information. The third unit is located in the frontal lobes and is responsible for programming, monitoring and verifying behaviour. Within the third unit, the prefrontal cortex is considered a superstructure and damage to this area in particular would lead to the disruption of complex behavioural programmes and a person's inability to regulate behaviour. More basic or stereotypical behaviours may result that are irrelevant, illogical or inappropriate (Chen *et al.* 2008).

Supervisory Attentional System

Norman and Shallice (1986) built upon Luria's original theory, with a focus on the third unit in particular, and developed the supervisory attentional system (SAS) (Figure 10.1).

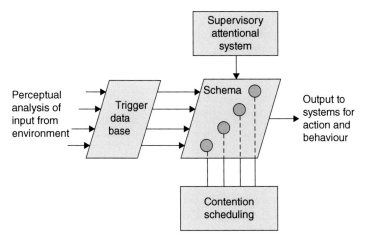

Figure 10.1 Diagram of Shallice model, the selection of action schemas. Source: Adapted from Shallice (1982).

According to this model, the prefrontal cortex, which is responsible for planning and regulating human behaviour, is thought to comprise two systems: contention scheduling and supervisory attentional. The former mediates routine, overlearned behaviours or activities such as making a cup of coffee. The latter is responsible for regulating non-routine or novel tasks such as preparing a new recipe.

Norman and Shallice named the following five situations in which contention scheduling would be insufficient for optimal performance, and the supervisory attentional would need to be activated:

- those that involve planning or decision making
- those that involve error detection or troubleshooting
- where responses are unique and need to be flexible
- where there is potential danger or risk
- those that require resisting temptation or overcoming a strong habitual response (Chen *et al.* 2008).

Stuss and Benson's Tripartite Model

Stuss and Benson (1986) posited that there are three systems that regulate attention and executive functions. The first and second, the anterior reticular activating system and the diffuse thalamic projection system, work together to maintain an individual's arousal and level of consciousness, as well as their level of alertness to external stimuli. The third system, known as the frontothalamic gating system, fulfils a similar role to the third unit described by Luria and the SAS described by Norman and Shallice. It is responsible for planning, response selection and monitoring of daily goal attainment and performance. However, the strength of this theory is based on how they expanded it to identify different attentional components of executive function at a neural level. These include:

- sustaining (right frontal)
- concentrating (cingulate area)
- sharing (cingulate and orbitofrontal area)

- suppressing (dorsolateral prefrontal cortex)
- switching (dorsolateral prefrontal and medial frontal areas)
- preparing (dorsolateral prefrontal cortex)
- goal setting (left dorsolateral prefrontal cortex) (Chen *et al.* 2008).

Damasio's Somatic Marker Hypothesis

Damasio (1995) developed a model to explain the 'hot' components of executive dysfunction and how they can affect the 'cold' components. It emphasises the role of the frontal lobe in emotion, social behaviour and decision making. According to Damasio, emotion is controlled by the prefrontal regions via complicated links between the cortex and subcortical regions. He proposed what he called a 'somatic hypothesis marker' to account for common impairments such as those seen with Phineas Gage, a railway construction worker in the nineteenth century who suffered severe damage to his ventromedial frontal cortex. He presented with a marked personality change, and had significant emotional and interpersonal problems. People with executive dysfunction may struggle to link inappropriate behaviours with an emotion-related somatic signal, leading to difficulties regulating their social behaviour (Bell 2006; Chen *et al.* 2008).

Routine and Non-Routine Behaviour

As mentioned above, Norman and Shallice (1986) developed the SAS model to explain the importance of differentiating between human behaviour in routine and novel situations. Executive dysfunction can affect behaviour in both, depending on its severity, but it is most apparent in non-routine circumstances when attention, working memory, insight and awareness need to be heightened to cope with the demands of initiating, goal setting, planning, organising, implementing, self-monitoring, problem solving and terminating a unique and unanticipated situation.

The SAS model identifies three different levels of executive functioning.

- Schema selection for a habitual action
- Contention scheduling to resolve conflict or inhibit competing schemas in schema selection
- Controlled processing of the SAS

To illustrate this, we will use the example of getting dressed in a suit for an important meeting at work. The subgoals of this activity are to select the needed items of clothing from the cupboard which include underwear, socks, belt, shirt, suit and tie. The next subgoal is to get dressed in the correct sequence so that trousers are not donned before underwear. Thus far, the schema selection for a habitual action will have been activated. However, whilst getting dressed, putting on jeans and a T-shirt which is far easier and more comfortable might be a temptation that would demand that contention scheduling is activated to inhibit this alternative schema from being initiated instead. Finally, if you discovered that your suit was in fact dirty, the SAS would need to be recruited to assist you to come up with an alternative solution for getting dressed. Perhaps you could borrow a suit from a friend, wear an alternative outfit of a shirt and smart trousers that would suffice, or get your suit dry cleaned in time for your afternoon meeting.

Metacognition

Metacognition is a broad term incorporating both knowledge and regulation of cognitive activity (Fernandez-Duque *et al.* 2000). Metacognitive knowledge is the knowledge people have about their cognitive skills (e.g. 'I can never concentrate for very long'), about cognitive strategies (e.g. 'To make sure I can focus on my work, I have to close my door and remove all distractions') and about tasks ('Visual information is easier for me to remember') (Fernandez-Duque *et al.* 2000). It has been called 'knowing what you know'.

Executive functions are inextricably linked with awareness in metacognition, with awareness as the more static component. Loss of awareness leads to the inability to detect errors in performance or to anticipate problems and plan strategies. Executive functions are dynamic and operate as a control system for self-monitoring and self-guidance.

Conceptual frameworks for metacognition, based on a hierarchy, have been developed (Katz and Hartman-Maeir 1997; Sohlberg *et al.* 1993) (Figure 10.2). Three levels are defined in the hierarchy and at each level, there is feedback down to the lower level.

- The lowest level is the cognitive skill for the acquisition and use of information from the environment in order to adapt to environmental demands. This level involves 'basic' cognitive skills, i.e. attention, perception and memory.
- The second level is the executive function for the formulation of realistic goals based on stored plans and routines, and for the development of strategies in flexible problem solving.
- The highest level is metacognitive skill for self-monitoring and self-correcting in the regulation of our actions and behaviour.

Figure 10.2 simply shows how metacognition comprises both the knowledge of one's cognition and the regulation of one's cognition.

Living with Executive Dysfunction

While understanding of the structure and neuroanatomical correlates of executive functions continues to evolve, there is broad agreement that executive dysfunction can have a debilitating effect on the lives of those affected and those close to them. The nature of the impairment also poses real challenges to rehabilitation therapists.

People with executive dysfunction tend to be forgetful, disorganised and unable to commence or complete tasks fully. They are easily distracted and poor at managing their time and their everyday activities. They are often unaware of the difficulties that they have and are reluctant to accept honest and direct feedback from family members and therapists, especially if they were competent and independent people prior to their injury or diagnosis. Such people may be able to intellectually verbalise their intentions and plans but are unable to execute them independently. Sometimes activities are not even initiated or if they are started, they are left unfinished because they are unable to break the tasks down into manageable parts, or because they are poor planners and use a disorganised approach. New situations are overwhelming and therefore avoided or inappropriately handled. The person may be apathetic or impulsive, easily angered or socially disinhibited; the box below details the lived experience.

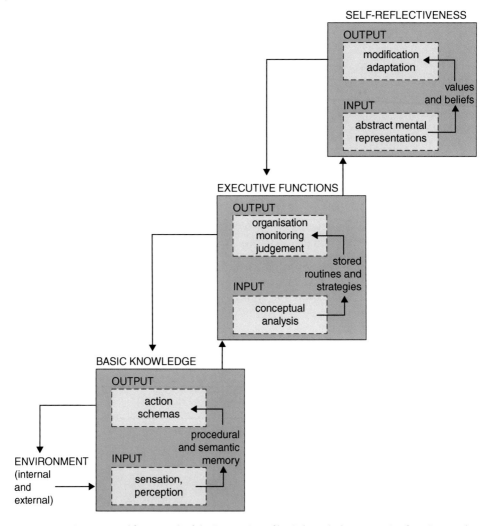

Figure 10.2 A conceptual framework of the interaction of basic knowledge, executive functions and self-reflectiveness. Source: Adapted from Sohlberg *et al.* (1993).

The lived experience of executive dysfunction, adapted from Headway (2013)

To start with, my girlfriend thought I was just being lazy; it's true that I have lost my 'get up and go'. I seem to be more impulsive now too; last week I bought a new television, as it was in the sale, but we didn't really need it. My parents say my mood swings are so difficult to cope with – I can be laughing out loud one minute and then crying the next. It makes it hard to socialise with my family and work colleagues; sometimes I just say the wrong thing at the wrong time.

My problems are not always noticeable to me but my girlfriend and mum tell me they are there; this can leave me feeling quite lonely and frustrated at times. But I'm learning to appreciate that my life problems are due to my brain injury and I'm starting to develop my own set of 'survival strategies'. I plan my week and do the same things on the same days; I use checklists for the simplest of things; when I am going out with my friends, I think about what I might need to avoid talking about so I don't put my foot in it.

I'm slowly adapting to my new brain; my smartphone has become essential for reminding me about things like appointments. And my family and friends have become even more important to me although I know they are also feeling the effects of living with this executive dysfunction.

Living with executive dysfunction can be extremely incapacitating, because normal life is filled with routine and novel encounters on a daily basis and to engage in all life's potential activities, we need the abilities and confidence to do so. Family and friends can provide a certain amount of support and assistance but also need their own support to understand and adapt to living with the person with executive dysfunction.

Suggestions for Assessment and Intervention

As outlined in Part 1 of this book, careful consideration must be given to the level of assessment we choose and the clinical reasoning behind our decisions. Body (or impairment) level tools may be required at the assessment stage but could be inappropriate as an outcome measure, given the persistence of executive dysfunction, as they would not capture improvements at the activity level.

It is also worth mentioning that depending on the severity of executive dysfunction, the person may perform well on standardised assessments whereas in fact they have great difficulty coping in day-to-day life.

Assessment

- Ensure your assessment considers the 'cold' and 'hot' components of executive function. 'Cold' components include abstract thinking, the ability to organise and plan, time management, cognitive flexibility, insight, judgement and problem solving (WHO 2001). 'Hot' components include interpersonal skills, social behaviour, personality and interpreting complex emotions (Chen *et al.* 2008; Damasio 1995).
- When selecting a tool or method, consider:
  - if you need to assess the actual impairment, for example to support clinical judgement if unsure of the presence of executive dysfunction
  - how you will assess the impact of executive dysfunction on carrying out daily activities
  - the importance of unstructured assessments to observe whether the person is able to structure and organise themselves
  - ways to include the family in the assessment process.
- Choose a multistep task that is novel but relevant to the person, and pitched at an appropriate level so that it is an achievable challenge for them to complete. Then use a non-standardised checklist approach, which questions the person and records performance of each component of the executive system as follows.
  - *Goal setting*: What do you intend to do? How long do you think it will take? How well do you think you will do on a scale of 1–10?

- *Planning*: What are all the steps involved in the activity?
- *Organising*: Do you have the equipment that you need? Do you need help from anyone else? Do you have enough time?
- *Initiation*: When will you begin the task?
- *Self-monitoring*: What problems may you encounter? What will you do if these arise?
- *Problem solving*: Can this task be done in more than one way?
- *Inhibition*: When will you know to stop the activity?

This approach, constructed by Ylvisacker and Szekeres (1989), can also be utilised as a method of intervention to assist people to self-question as they perform non-routine activities.

Assessment Resources

Body level assessment tools include the Hayling Sentence Completion Test (Chen *et al.* 2008) for the assessment of verbal initiation and inhibition, the Brixton Spatial Anticipation Test (Chen *et al.* 2008) for the assessment of rule detection and impulsivity, and the Behavioural Assessment of Dysexecutive Syndrome (BADS) (Wilson *et al.* 1996) for the assessment of temporal awareness, problem solving, switching, planning, strategy allocation and self-monitoring.

Resources that assess activity and participation include the Assessment of Motor and Process Skills (AMPS) and the Dysexecutive Questionnaire (Wilson *et al.* 1996) for the assessment of behaviours associated with intentionality, inhibition, executive memory, and positive and negative affect. The latter is a 20-item questionnaire to be completed by the person with executive dysfunction and a person close to them.

Intervention

- Establish *structure* with the person in their daily routine, preferably in collaboration with those close to them. Structure can be enhanced through the use of a range of external aids and internal strategies.
- Educate the person on executive functions and the associated impairments, as this may improve self-awareness and motivation to participate in therapy proactively.
- Educate family members on the nature of the impairment and the impact of it on daily life as this may increase their understanding of executive dysfunction as a consequence of the health condition.
- *Goal management training (GMT)* – GMT is specifically designed for people with executive dysfunction and is divided into five stages. 1. Stop and ask 'What am I doing?'. 2. Define the main goal or task at hand. 3. List the steps to complete the task. 4. Learn the steps. 5. Check and ask 'Am I doing what I planned to do?' (Levine *et al.* 2000).
- *Short-Term Executive Plus (STEP)* – this is a specialised, novel and intensive programme. The goal is to teach a set of metacognitive skills that can be applied across a wide range of real-life activities. The treatments included in STEP are problem-solving training, emotional regulation training, attention training and use of cognitive supports. It is intended to run over a period of 12 weeks and includes group therapy that focuses on problem solving and emotional regulation, and individual therapy focusing on attention and compensatory strategies (Cantor *et al.* 2014).

SUMMARY

1) Executive functions are composed of a number of higher order cognitive skills that need to work together to enable a person to function at the highest level. The component skills include initiation, inhibition, goal setting and intentionality, planning and organising, self-monitoring and problem solving. All of these utilise the more fundamental skills of attention, working memory and self-awareness to optimise everyday function.
2) Executive dysfunction can occur following a range of injuries and conditions affecting the brain. The prefrontal cortex plays a pivotal role but other subcortical areas are also involved. Traumatic brain injury is the most common cause but stroke, Parkinson's disease, Alzheimer's disease, schizophrenia and depression are a few of numerous others that can also result in executive dysfunction.
3) There are a number of models and theories to explain executive function, and a host of assessment tools to assist with its accurate diagnosis when it is impaired. People living with executive dysfunction experience significant difficulty in living independently, returning to work/school/study and maintaining relationships.
4) Compensatory interventions are required to help a person and their family to adapt and make the changes in their daily lives, through the implementation of structure, education, self-awareness training, memory and attention training and goal management training in the context of their home and work environments. Engaging with family members and others close to the person is crucial as part of learning to develop 'survival strategies' and adapt to life with executive dysfunction.

References

Andres, P. and van der Linden, M. (2000) Age-related differences in supervisory attentional system functions. *Journal of Gerontology:Psychological Sciences*, **55B** (6), 373–380.

Bell, V. (2006) The executive system and its disorders. www.ldchicago.com/execsysdisorders.pdf (accessed 28 September 2016).

Burgess, P., Alderman, N., Evans, J., Emslie, H. and Wilson, B. (1998) The ecological validity of tests of executive function. *Journal of the International Neuropsychological Society*, **4**, 547–558.

Cantor, J., Ashman, T., Dams-O'Connor, K. *et al.* (2014) Evaluation of the STEP intervention for executive dysfunction after traumatic brain injury: a randomized controlled trial with minimization. *Archives of Physical Medicine and Rehabilitation*, **95**, 1–9.

Chen, R., Shum, D., Toulopoulou, T. and Chen E. (2008) Assessment of executive functions: review of instruments and identification of critical issues. *Archives of Clinical Neuropsychology*, **23**, 201–216.

Chung, C., Pollock, A., Campbell, T., Durward, B. and Hagan, S. (2013) Cognitive rehabilitation for executive dysfunction in adults with stroke or other adult non-progressive acquired brain damage. *Stroke*, **44**, e77–e78.

Damasio, A.R. (1994) *Descartes's Error: Emotion, Reason and the Human Brain*. G.P. Putnam, New York.

Damasio, A.R. (1995) Toward a neurobiology of emotion and feeling: Operational concepts and hypotheses. *The Neuroscientist*, **1** (1), 19–25.

Elliot, R. (2003) Executive functions and their disorders. *British Medical Bulletin*, **65**, 49–59.

Fernandez-Duque, D., Baird, J. and Posner, M. (2000) Executive attention and metacognitive regulation. *Consciousness and Cognition*, **9**, 288–307.

Headway (2013) Executive dysfunction after brain injury. Available at: www.headway.org. uk/executive-dysfunction-after-brain-injury.aspx (accessed 26 September 2016).

Katz, N. and Hartman-Maeir, A. (1997) Occupational performance and metacognition. *Canadian Journal of Occupational Therapy*, **64** (2), 53–62.

Levine, B., Robertson, I., Clare, L. *et al.* (2000) Rehabilitation of executive functioning: an experimental-clinical validation of goal management training. *Journal of the International Neuropsychological Society*, **6**, 299–312.

Luria, A.R. (1966) *The Higher Cortical Functions in Man*. Basic Books, New York.

Norman, D.A., and Shallice, T., (1986) *Attention to action. In Consciousness and self-regulation* (pp. 1–18). Springer US.

Novakovic-Agopian, T., Chen, A., Rome, S. *et al.* (2011) Rehabilitation of executive functioning with training in attention regulation applied to individually defined goals: a pilot study bridging theory, assessment and treatment. *Journal of Head Trauma and Rehabilitation*, **26** (5), 325–338.

Shallice, T. (1982) Specific impairment of planning. *Philosophical Transactions of the Royal Society of London B*, **298**, 199–209.

Sohlberg, M.M., Mateer, C. and Stuss, D.T. (1993) Contemporary approaches to the management of executive control dysfunction. *Journal of Head Trauma Rehabilitation*, **8** (1), 45–58.

Stuss, D. and Alexander, M. (2000) Executive functions and the frontal lobes: a conceptual view. *Psychological Research*, **63**, 289–298.

Stuss, D.T., and Benson, D.F. (1986) *The frontal lobes*, Raven Press, New York.

Wilson, B., Alderman N., Burgess P., Emslie. H. and Evans, J. (1996) *Behavioural Assessment of the Dysexecutive Syndrome (BADS)*, Thames Valley Test Company, Bury St Edmunds.

World Health Organisation (2001) *International Classification of Functioning, Disability and Health (ICF)*. World Health Organisation, Geneva.

Ylvisacker, M. & Szekeres, S.F. (1989) Metacognitive and executive impairments in head-injured children and adults. *Topics in Language Disorders*, **9** (2), 34–49.

11

Cognitive Function in the General Population

Maintaining Cognitive Health in Later Years

Linda Maskill

AIMS

1) To take a wider perspective of cognitive functioning as a whole with a focus upon later life, and position this within the context of threats to cognitive health relating to lifestyle and ageing in societies across the globe.
2) To introduce mild cognitive impairment (MCI) as a concept and emerging health concern due to its impact upon occupation and its relationship to dementia.
3) To identify MCI, multimorbidity and frailty as interrelated conditions comprising a triad of health issues affecting older people.
4) To explore the evidence for occupationally focused strategies and approaches to working with all service user populations and the general public, to:
   - maintain health and minimise risks for the development of MCI
   - support cognitive function and occupational well-being in later years.
5) To consider the development of occupational therapy provision for people with MCI.

Introduction and Rationale

This chapter is a new addition to *Neuropsychology for Occupational Therapists*. Positioned as the last chapter of the book, it departs from the design of the preceding chapters, which focused on specific cognitive functions and assessment and interventions for clinically diagnosed or recognised impairments. This chapter addresses the need for a holistic, preventive approach in light of emerging knowledge of general cognitive health and impairment as it affects the older population.

The rationale for this chapter is derived from current and emerging concerns about demographic change and the health needs associated with populations living longer into old age. In 2000, the percentage of the population in Europe aged 60 and over was 20%.

Neuropsychology for Occupational Therapists: Cognition in Occupational Performance, Fourth Edition.
Edited by Linda Maskill and Stephanie Tempest.
© 2017 John Wiley & Sons Ltd. Published 2017 by John Wiley & Sons Ltd.
Companion Website: www.wiley.com/go/maskill/neuropsychologyOT

> The total cost of dementia to society in the UK is £26.3 billion, with an average cost of £32,250 per person.
> - £4.3 billion is spent on healthcare costs.
> - £10.3 billion is spent on social care (publicly and privately funded).
> - £11.6 billion is contributed by the work of unpaid carers of people with dementia.

Figure 11.1 The cost of dementia in the UK. Source: Prince *et al.* (2014).

By 2050 it is predicted to rise to 35%. Worldwide, in the same time-span, the 60+ population is predicted to grow from around 10% (606 million) to around 20% (2 billion) (Butler *et al.* 2004). In the UK, as elsewhere, this has raised concerns about the capacity of health and welfare services to respond to need and provide interventions, care and support to ageing populations. This is compounded by the shift in age distribution, such that the concern is not only the number of older people who may be in need of care but also the relatively smaller numbers of younger adults of working age required to generate an economy to support the predicted costs, or indeed to provide that care. Figure 11.1 gives the cost breakdown for dementia care in the UK.

A critical factor in what degree of societal and economic 'burden' an ageing population may become is the difference between healthy life expectancy and overall life expectancy. That is, the time from when a person is no longer able to function independently and starts requiring support or care until death. Some estimates put this figure at an average of 10 years in developed societies (King's Fund 2015), and it follows that if this time period can be reduced (by increasing healthy life expectancy) then the social and economic costs of old age can be reduced and quality of life maintained for longer.

Dementia is the predominant manifestation of cognition-related disability and high-level dependency in old age. Its current and predicted prevalence make it a significant determinant of care and support needs, and a major factor in the healthy versus overall life expectancy time gap. By addressing the precursors of this condition and factors implicated in their development, preventive interventions may play a meaningful role in reducing disability and dependency, and extending healthy life expectancy.

The Growing Prevalence of Dementia: Inevitable or Not?

It is estimated that currently, in the UK, 1 in 14 people aged 65 and over has dementia. Late-onset (after the age of 65) dementia accounts for the majority of cases (95%), while the prevalence in people aged 60–64 is estimated at 0.9% – nearly 1 in 100. Assuming that prevalence remains stable (i.e. no major changes occur in risk factors or causation) then demographic changes alone will drive increases as demographic shifts towards an older population continue (Prince *et al.* 2014). Other factors come into play, some pushing towards an increase in prevalence, others militating against. Better education, better control of cardiovascular diseases and reductions in smoking, heart disease and stroke, and successful public health initiatives militate for a decrease in prevalence. Increases in and earlier onset of type 2 diabetes, a rise in obesity and physical inactivity, and improved survival rates after stroke and in vascular conditions are factors that may push a rise in prevalence. Overall, there is some evidence in developed countries that the factors that decrease prevalence may be outweighing those that increase it, and that people may still develop dementia but its onset is occurring later. This brings us back to the issue of healthy versus overall life expectancy, indicating that the gap in between may be shortening in some areas of the world. However, in some developing countries, risk factors are increasing, including stroke, ischaemic heart disease, obesity and hypertension (Prince *et al.* 2014).

All these risk factors arguably have one thing in common – they are largely preventable or at least modifiable through lifestyle and behavioural change, through how people construct and conduct their activities and occupations. This is underlined by the Alzheimer's Society's (UK) assertion that the worst case scenario can be expected if current, early improvements in public health do not continue, i.e. health and social care services will not be able to cope, and family and informal carers will be increasingly left to struggle to provide care.

Mild Cognitive Impairment

The concept of mild cognitive impairment (MCI) has developed over the last few decades, as awareness has grown of the existence of a 'grey area' in which mild cognitive changes are present in a proportion of the older population but are not of sufficient significance clinically or functionally to meet the criteria for a diagnosis of dementia. The progression rate to dementia from MCI has been given as 5–15% per year compared to 1–6% per year in people without MCI.

Initially conceived as a predementia state, requiring the presence of memory impairments, research has subsequently identified that MCI is not always a precursor to dementia, and could affect domains of cognitive function other than memory. The most recent definition of MCI recognises four key criteria for a diagnosis to be established: self- or informant-reported cognitive complaint, presence of an objective cognitive impairment, preserved independence in functional abilities and no dementia (Petersen *et al.* 2014). MCI is further classified as amnestic (aMCI), if memory is impaired with or without impairment in other cognitive domains, or non-amnestic (naMCI) if there is no memory impairment. It can further be differentiated according to the number of cognitive domains affected, as either single or multi-domain (sdMCI or mdMCI) (Petersen *et al.* 2014; Sachdev *et al.* 2012) (Figure 11.2).

MCI and Mild Neurocognitive Disorder

The latest version of the *Diagnostic and Statistical Manual of Mental Disorders* (DSM-5) (American Psychiatric Association 2013) introduced a new diagnostic category, for the first time, of mild neurocognitive disorder (mNCD) as distinct from major NCDs (such as dementia), that may progress to dementia or may not. It has parallels to MCI and is defined as an identifiable decrement in cognitive functioning requiring some adjustments in order to maintain independence and carry out activities of daily living (ADL), but not interfering with independence. The virtues of a standardised definition and classification include recommendations on the use of objective methods of assessment, early identification enabling implementation of preventive strategies and support to the individual for management and future planning (Sachs-Ericsson and Blazer 2015). It is possible, if not likely, that mNCD may supersede MCI as the favoured term for this group of mild cognitive disorders, bringing with it a degree of clarity and recognition and a framework for approach.

Defining features of MCI
- Cognitive complaint reported by self or other
- Presence of objective cognitive impairment
- Preserved independence in activities of daily living
- No dementia

MCI subtypes

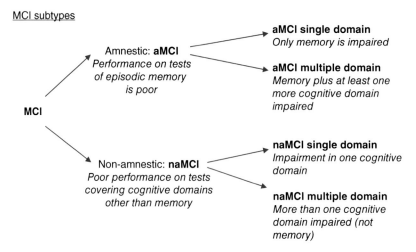

Figure 11.2 Defining features and subtypes of MCI. Source: Petersen *et al.* (2014).

Risk Factors for MCI and Associated Conditions

Research into MCI prevalence and the risk factors associated with its development is still in its early stages. In the last 15 years, a number of studies (see Petersen *et al.* 2014, Table 3) conducted across the world have produced prevalence estimates for MCI in the general population aged 65+ with a mean of 18.9%. That is approaching 1 in 5 older people. Studies have explored the association between cognitive function in later years and nutrition, obesity, smoking, diabetes, cardiovascular health, social engagement, physical activity and aerobic fitness. Several observational cohort studies have followed people during old age and from early or mid-adulthood into old age, while a growing number of intervention-control studies seek to manipulate key variables (such as physical activity) and measure changes in cognitive function and other aspects of health. While these studies vary in size and some findings are inconsistent, a general picture is emerging of risk factors for, and protective factors against, the development and progression of MCI and/or dementia. Table 11.1 provides a selection of studies and their key findings. In short, convincing evidence is accumulating for the role of physical health, nutrition, social engagement and cardiovascular fitness as modifiable factors influencing the maintenance or decline of cognitive health and capacity in old age and the development of MCI.

Frailty

Frailty is a clinical condition incorporating multiple functional and physiological features in which homeostatic mechanisms, and the ability to withstand or recover from stressors, are severely compromised. It is age related and highly associated with

Table 11.1 Selected studies for risk and preventive factors in cognitive health and function in older adults.

Authors	Study	Findings
Barnes *et al.* 2004	Relationship between social resources and cognitive decline in older adults. Data from the Chicago Health and Aging Project. 6102 subjects	Higher number of social networks and level of social engagement correlated positively with initial level of cognitive function and both were associated with a reduced rate of cognitive decline
Haslam *et al.* 2014	Evidence for the distinctive benefits of group engagement in enhancing cognitive health in aging. Data from the English Longitudinal Study of Ageing. 3413 subjects	Comparison of engagement in group vs individual social activities showed that only group engagement made a significant and sustained contribution to subsequent cognitive function. Group engagement optimised health outcomes, especially with increasing age
Hotting and Roder 2013	Review of evidence for the effects of physical exercise on neuroplasticity and cognition, in humans at different ages and across the lifespan	Physical exercise may trigger processes facilitating neuroplasticity, enhancing capacity to respond and adapt to new demands and mechanisms underlying brain health and function. Combining physical and cognitive training may further enhance outcomes. To maintain benefits, the level of cardiovascular fitness may need to be maintained
Tournoy *et al.* 2010	Association of cognitive performance with the metabolic syndrome (MetS) and glycaemia in middle-aged and older European men: the European Male Ageing Study. 3152 subjects with complete data	Men without MetS performed better on all cognitive tests compared with men who had MetS. However, the syndrome was not associated with cognitive impairment, but analysis of individual factors showed an inverse association between blood glucose levels and cognitive performance. Men with diabetes had (significantly) the lowest scores
Wendell *et al.* 2009	Carotid intimal medial thickness (IMT) as a measure of subclinical vascular disease and its relationship to cognitive decline in adults without clinical vascular disease. The Baltimore Longitudinal Study of Ageing. 538 subjects	Individuals with greater carotid IMT showed accelerated decline in performance on a number of tests of cognition over time. Carotid IMT predicts accelerated cognitive decline in individuals free of vascular and neurological disease
Wendell *et al.* 2014	Prospective study of adults aged 19–94 over 18 years, measuring cardiorespiratory fitness by maximal oxygen consumption (VO_{2max}) and comparing with performance on tests of cognition. Baltimore Longitudinal Study of Aging. 615 subjects	Individuals (aged 50+) with reduced VO_{2max} at baseline showed greater prospective decline in performance on multiple measures of memory and a cognitive screening tool. Poorer fitness was associated with accelerated memory decline, greater fitness with less decline across the lifespan

(Continued)

Table 11.1 (Continued)

Authors	Study	Findings
Wennberg *et al.* 2014	Diabetes and cognitive outcomes in a nationally representative sample: the National Health and Aging Trends Study (USA). 7606 subjects	Type 2 diabetes mellitus was associated with poorer cognitive test performance on immediate and delayed word recall, and poorer self-rated memory
Wilson *et al.* 2014	Relationship between 25-hydroxyvitamin D and cognitive function in older adults: the Health, Ageing and Body Composition Study (Health ABC). 2777 subjects	Low levels of 25(OH)D were associated with worse global cognitive decline over time

adverse health outcomes (Buchman *et al.* 2007; Clegg *et al.* 2013). Only in the last decade or so has it become recognised and established as a distinct syndrome, characterised by a decrease in reserve and homeostatic resilience across several physiological systems. A diagnosis of frailty does not require the pre-existence of any specific health condition, as it is considered a distinct clinical syndrome, but frequently occurs in association with one or more other chronic conditions (cardiac, neurological, musculoskeletal) and with disability.

There are a range of elements that combine to generate frailty, and a number of models and associated measures have been developed for its identification, with considerable overlap. In brief, frailty may be indicated by a combination of presenting factors such as weight loss, self-reported exhaustion, slow gait speed, weak grip strength, very low energy expenditure and/or the presence of a number of more specific impairments such as tremor, low mood or disability.

Although considered a condition affecting a minority of older people, prevalence within the community has been estimated at 10% of all over-65 s, with an increase to 26% or more in those over 85 (Clegg *et al.* 2013). Frailty *per se* substantially increases risks for health and independence and, with a growth in population ageing, will contribute significantly to increasing demands upon health and social care services.

Studies are emerging that have identified an association between frailty and cognitive decline. In a 12-year study by Boyle *et al.* (2010) of 760 people, 40% developed MCI. By measuring frailty over the same period, they found that each unit increase in frailty was associated with a 63% increase in MCI, and that higher levels of frailty were associated with a faster rate of decline in cognitive functions.

Multimorbidity, Frailty and MCI

Multimorbidity is common with increasing age and, like frailty, is associated with loss of functional independence, increased use of health and social care services and poor outcomes. In a study that analysed a large dataset of people registered with primary care practices in Scotland, Barnett *et al.* (2012) found that 23% of patients had multimorbidity (i.e. two or more concurrent chronic conditions) overall, and that by age 65, more than 50% were multimorbid, rising to 75% by age 84. In effect, multimorbidity is the norm rather than the exception within the general older population.

There is limited evidence identifying associations between MCI and physical multi-morbidity *per se*, but studies have measured the presence of MCI in populations with specific chronic conditions, exploring its association with adverse outcomes. In turn, specific chronic conditions have been explored in terms of coincident morbidities of frailty and MCI. Three examples follow as illustrations.

- Partridge *et al.* (2014) investigated the prevalence of undiagnosed cognitive impairment in older people presenting for vascular surgery to a UK hospital. They found that 77 (68%) patients had MCI or dementia, previously unrecognised in 68 of them, therefore 60% of their surgical patients had non-diagnosed cognitive impairment. They also found that a score denoting impairment on a cognitive test was strongly associated with pre-existing frailty. The combination of cognitive impairment with frailty was strongly predictive of adverse outcomes and longer hospital stay.
- Using 1927 participants enrolled in the Mayo Clinic Study of Aging (USA), Singh *et al.* (2013) found that patients with chronic obstructive pulmonary disease (COPD) had a higher prevalence of MCI than those without (27% as opposed to 15%).
- Park *et al.* (2013), using data from a national health and nutrition dataset in North America, found that in a sample of 211 people diagnosed with COPD, emphysema or chronic bronchitis, 21.8% were prefrail and 57.8% (122) were frail. Impaired cognition was found in 19.9% or 42 people.

In summary, we find that multimorbidities, including frailty, are common in older age and together with MCI, probably form an underestimated triad of factors that undermine the health and independent function of significant numbers of older people. That frailty predicts MCI and cognitive decline has implications for public health. That frailty and co-morbidities are serious threats to the health and independence of older people, and both have high associations with the development of MCI, reinforces the importance of health promotion and preventive interventions – the need to develop public health strategies that support the maintenance of cognitive health, physical health and vitality across the life course.

The Impact of MCI on Function

A diagnosis of MCI as currently defined (Petersen *et al.* 2014) requires that although there are measurable changes in cognitive functioning, the person remains independent in the performance of ADL. Similarly, the DSM-V criteria for diagnosis of mNCD require that independence in ADL is not affected, but does identify that performance may require more effort or that (behavioural) adaptations are used to complete activities (American Psychiatric Association 2013). However, there is clear evidence that MCI does affect functional activity performance, and that this typically involves the more complex ADLs that require higher cognitive effort (Puente *et al.* 2014; Reppermund *et al.* 2013). These activities fall within the occupational construct of instrumental ADL (IADL), and include management of finances, shopping, cooking and driving. Some authors further differentiate the most complex IADL as advanced or a-ADL. These may include driving, use of technology and travelling, i.e. activities that go beyond those necessary to live independently (de Vriendt *et al.* 2013).

IADL Performance as an Indicator of MCI

To date, the retention of independence in ADL has probably been a significant factor precluding consideration of need by people with MCI for therapeutic occupational intervention. Occupational therapists are mostly involved with people who demonstrate significant functional and behavioural change (i.e. those with dementias) and where interventions may promote retention of independence, safety and the skills needed for basic ADL. Service priorities and resourcing issues generally preclude consideration of or intervention for aspects of daily life that might be considered non-essential. However, evidence is growing not only for a greater impact of MCI upon IADL than previously thought, but also for the potential use of objective IADL measures to detect early cognitive decline. Both of these developments begin to establish a basis of need for occupational therapy services to the MCI population.

Rodakowski *et al.* (2014) have shown that assessment of cognitively focused IADL (e.g. shopping, bill paying, chequebook balancing) can discriminate between older adults with cognitively normal function and those with MCI. They assessed 96 cognitively normal and 61 mildly cognitive impaired older adults in performance on eight activities, using the Performance Assessment of Self-Care Skills (PASS) (Rodakowski *et al.* 2014). They found that those with MCI displayed more preclinical disability, and that such disability was possibly more pronounced than had hitherto been thought. Furthermore, their work suggested that the scores on the IADL tasks could be more accurate in classifying cognitive status than scores on a standard and widely used test of cognitive function, the Mini-Mental State Examination (MMSE).

Puente *et al.* (2014) compared the basic and instrumental ADL performance of 20 cognitively normal older adults, with 30 who had a diagnosis of MCI. For assessment of ADL, they used a self-report measure, a collateral report questionnaire (completed by another who had regular close contact) and an objective performance-based measure – the DAFS-R (McDougall *et al.* 2010). No significant differences were found between the groups on the self- and other-report measures, but significant differences occurred for IADL tasks on the performance-based measure. No differences were found between the groups on performance of basic ADL. This adds further to the evidence for need of objective functional assessment, and to the impact of MCI on performance of cognitively more demanding activities.

Maintaining Cognitive Health and Preventing Decline: The Role of Occupations

Chronic, often lifestyle-associated health conditions have replaced infectious disease and trauma as major sources of ill health and disability for older people in developed and developing societies. For many, chronic disease, multimorbidity and frailty mark old age, generating loss of independence and a need for increased health provision and care in the years, often decades, leading to the end of life. Prince *et al.* (2014) suggest that efforts to effect lifestyle change through public health and education may have the greatest positive impact upon people currently in their 30s and 40s. Not only would this confer greatest benefit, building biological and cognitive 'capital' for good health and homeostatic resilience in old age, but it would enable them to influence the health of the next generation to whom they are parents and educators.

Consensus exists that the ageing process operates from the very beginning of life; what occurs *in utero*, during early years and onwards influences health and vulnerability to chronic diseases in later life. While genetics account significantly for predisposition and disease development, modifiable factors and chance events wield substantial influence over risk factors and probabilities, and make a critical contribution to the 'biological capital' we have, or don't have, available to withstand threats to health. Hence, a 'life-course' approach to ageing and health is recognised as necessary to underpin health promotion, disease prevention, and management of ill health, through childhood into adulthood and old age (Kuh 2007). There is a growing understanding of this complex interplay of modifiable and non-modifiable factors over time and their contribution to healthy and overall life expectancy. Biological capital, and the need to build, maintain or restore it, is recognised as a critical concept underpinning non-medical health interventions, whether preventive, remediative or compensatory.

Against this background, research is providing increasing evidence for lifestyle and other factors that promote good health and reduce risks of chronic disease and cognitive decline, and may prevent or slow the onset of substantial ill health and disability. What these factors have in common is that they are elements of daily life that, by their absence or presence and their frequency of being practised and incorporated into routine, influence body function, mental and physical capacity, vulnerability and resilience. Research is also highlighting that essentially, what is good for body is also good for mind, and that interventions designed to address aspects of physical health confer cognitive benefits, and vice versa. Activities of daily living, our occupations and how they are practised, are the key components.

Evidence for Preventive Action

Table 11.1 highlighted some studies where evidence was found for the beneficial effects on cognitive function of social engagement, physical exercise and physical fitness. Nutrition, weight and glucose metabolism, cardiovascular fitness, cognitive challenge, general activity levels, tobacco use and alcohol intake are also modifiable factors that appear to influence physiological processes at system and cellular level, contributing to brain health. The effects of tobacco and alcohol are generally well recognised. Below we consider some of the evidence for the role of diet and weight management, physical fitness and cardiovascular status in cognitive health.

The relative recency of research into MCI means that the majority of evidence for relationships between interventions and prevention discusses effectiveness in terms of dementia risk or progression. The UK Department of Health report on physical activity for health (DoH 2011) identified evidence for a clear relationship between physical activity levels and the prevention of depression and dementia, although no evidence for a dose–response relationship existed. The Department of Health report considers that any amount of physical activity can confer benefits to both physical and cognitive health, but the recommended minimum for all adults to aim for is 150 minutes of moderate to intense physical activity per week, distributed across the week. The report recognises that most older people obtain physical exercise because it forms a component of routine daily activity, and recommends meaningful activities as media through which to achieve targets, for example leisure interests such as bowls, walking or swimming or

Table 11.2 Percentages of the UK population achieving minimum recommended physical activity levels: self-report data. Source: Based on DoH (2011).

Country	Men	Women	Boys	Girls
England	40%	28%	32%	24%
Northern Ireland	33%	28%	19%	10%
Wales	36%	23%	63%	45%
Scotland	43%	32%	76%	67%
UK overall averages	**38%**	**28%**	**47.5%**	**36.5%**

as a part of necessary tasks such as shopping and housework. This supports the argument that occupations, and the contexts of their performance, are keys to achieving and maintaining beneficial physical activity and therefore cognitive health.

The major and critical concern for adults of all ages, and children, is that the majority fail to meet even minimum recommended activity levels. Table 11.2 shows the percentages in the UK achieving these levels, based largely on self-report evidence. However, objective studies using accelerometry suggest that the percentages for adults are even lower – 6% for men and 4% for women (DoH 2011). It is also known that levels of physical activity decline with age, so that by age 75, only 9% of men and 5% of women achieve minimum recommended levels.

In addition to the need for physical activity and fitness, nutrition and weight management have received increasing attention as factors in maintaining general health and preventing the development of chronic diseases. Obesity is associated with increased risk of cardiovascular disease, type 2 diabetes, degenerative arthritis and some cancers. Diabetes and cardiovascular disease are risk factors for cognitive impairment and dementia. The prevalence of obesity and type 2 diabetes is rising not only in middle-aged and older adults, but worryingly so in young adults and children. This is clearly linked to diet and sedentary activity. Excessive intake of simple and refined carbohydrates and saturated fats appears to be a critical factor in their effects upon metabolic activity at cellular level. It can be argued that lack of physical activity to drive energy use and regulate hormonal and other homeostatic processes also plays a part in this.

Physiologically, these factors appear to operate by inducing adverse changes in cell function and survival. Such change is thought to underlie pathological brain ageing and cognitive decline (Bishop *et al.* 2010; Cholerton *et al.* 2011; Kanoski and Davidson 2011). Other models that offer explanations for the link between diet and cognitive deterioration consider that impaired glucose regulation and metabolic syndrome (where a person exhibits three or more of abdominal obesity, hypertension, hyperlipidaemia, high fasting glucose and high triglycerides) contribute to impairment of vascular reactivity, neuroinflammation, oxidative stress and abnormal brain lipid metabolism (Yates *et al.* 2012).

This evidence, and the established associations between obesity, excess carbohydrate intake, dietary deficiencies (such as vitamin D, calcium) and chronic health conditions, reinforces the importance of nutritional education and guidance at all ages. Again, cognitive health becomes an issue of daily activities and occupational considerations, this time in relation to food selection, preparation and consumption.

Direct relationships have been found between measures of cardiovascular health and cognitive function. A study by Wendell *et al.* (2009) measured carotid artery intimal media thickness and performance on a range of cognitive tests. Subjects were aged 20–93 years and were without any clinical vascular disease. The study found clear inverse relationships between intimal media thickness and cognitive performance, such that greater thickness was significantly associated with poorer performance on a number of measures. They also found that individuals with greater intimal media thickness showed accelerated decline over time. In research drawing upon the same long-term prospective study (from the Baltimore Longitudinal Study of Aging), Wendell *et al.* (2014) compared VO_{2max} (a measure of cardiorespiratory fitness) with performance on a battery of neuropsychological tests. They found that cognitive function was positively associated with cardiorespiratory fitness, that those with higher VO_{2max} performed better on the tests, and also that those with higher VO_{2max} over time showed a slower decline on the tests.

Studies examining the relationship between aerobic exercise and cognitive function, and effects of exercise on brain volume, have produced promising results. In brief, consistent findings support the beneficial effects of aerobic fitness training on brain health. Colcombe *et al.* (2006) found significant increases in brain volume, in both grey and white matter regions, in older people who participated in aerobic training but not for those who undertook non-aerobic training. Brinke *et al.* (2015) demonstrated that aerobic exercise can increase hippocampal volume in a small sample of older women with MCI, although this did not translate into better performance on cognitive testing. Barber *et al.* (2012) summarised the neuroprotective effects of exercise training – that it has been shown to increase the activity of several neurotrophic and vascular growth factors and upregulate the functions they mediate, including neurogenesis, synaptic plasticity and angiogenesis.

Finally, a meta-analytic study by Colcombe and Kramer (2003) found unequivocal evidence that aerobic fitness training has robust and beneficial effects upon cognitive function in sedentary older adults. Executive functions showed the greatest overall benefit, but overlapping visuospatial functions also showed some benefit. In general, it appeared that those processes and functions most severely affected by cognitive decline were the functions that seemed to benefit most from aerobic fitness training. It is hard to deny that inclusion of physical exercise, with an emphasis upon aerobic activities, is important in daily activities and as part of an individual's occupational profile, if cognitive health and function are to be maintained.

Is There a Need for Occupational Therapy?

In summary, the evidence for maintenance of cognitive health and prevention of decline supports an emphasis upon incorporation of beneficial practices (habits and routine) within personal and instrumental activities of daily living, and educational, productive and leisure occupations. A life-course approach is needed, with public health and education directed to supporting people of all ages to acquire and adopt healthy lifestyle practices. It is clear that age is not a barrier to improving health or to implementing strategies to maintain cognitive health. It is equally clear that daily activities are the medium through which lifestyle change can be effected.

The many lifestyle factors that increase risk of cognitive decline and chronic ill health are ubiquitous, and therefore opportunities to enable and facilitate maintenance and prevention need to be equally ubiquitous. Affluence, technology, changing work and leisure habits, amongst others, have substantially changed lifestyles, for example reducing the need for physical effort in many aspects of daily life or making poor food choices difficult to avoid or resist. Many people are at risk – figures for prevalence of MCI and associated chronic health conditions bear that out – and it follows therefore that health professionals, including occupational therapists, are well placed to drive health promotion for the prevention of cognitive decline, as well as having an obligation to do so. The key objectives in such a preventive strategy include the following.

- Incorporation of physical activity into daily and weekly routine – at all ages, aiming for recommended levels of moderate to intense aerobic exercise with maintenance of optimal fitness.
- Attention to calorie intake and nutritional quality of food.
- Maintenance of a healthy weight.
- Engagement in meaningful group social activities.
- Smoking cessation and moderation of alcohol intake.

Making Every Contact Count – Promoting Good Physical and Mental Health

In 2012, the NHS Future Forum produced a report into the role of the NHS in the UK public's health. This document identified the role that lifestyle, nutrition, physical inactivity and socioeconomic factors play in the development and prevalence of chronic ill health in the general population, and set out the principles and priorities for action to improve health and well-being. This introduced the concept of 'Making Every Contact Count' (MECC), and identified that it was the responsibility of every health and social care service, and their employees, to use every contact with the individuals they worked with to improve and maintain their physical and mental health, even if only by encouraging a small change. It was recommended that this approach should be incorporated into the NHS Constitution, and that all staff should receive training and support to implement health promotion activities. Critical to its implementation and sustainability was that it should not increase workload, but form a part of day-to-day business and practice. Another key feature was the recognition that staff need to be trained and supported not only in helping their clients and patients to make change, but also to be able to change their own behaviours and improve their own health – that the NHS should 'put its own house in order' if it expected its users to do the same (NHS Future Forum 2012).

Although not aimed specifically at prevention of MCI, the four key health issues targeted by MECC are all implicated as major modifiable risk factors for its development: tobacco smoking, alcohol consumption, diet and physical activity. Therefore, engaging with and implementing the MECC approach has the potential to reduce the incidence of MCI. It is becoming an obligation of all health professionals in the UK to adopt MECC, and a requirement of leaders and managers of services to support staff in improving their own health and to enable this approach.

Two initiatives provide examples of how MECC is being promoted by services and health professional organisations.

- Percival (2014) reported on a training programme devised under the auspices of the Royal College of Nursing, to support the determination that every nurse interaction with a patient should be seen as an opportunity to promote good health and prevent illness.
- An implementation guide and toolkit for MECC has been developed by the East Midlands Trainer Hub (NHS) (undated) and made available free of charge online for all health and social care organisations to make use of, including a range of resources. This addresses the responsibilities and actions required of organisations and their employees to achieve systematic and sustainable change to support implementation of MECC.

It is expected that over time, more UK organisations and services will engage with MECC and develop educational and training programmes for their employees and members.

Interventions for MCI

Action may be targeted not just at helping people to avoid onset of MCI, but also at slowing or halting deterioration, or even reversing decline. Drug interventions have not as yet shown efficacy, and therefore the emphasis remains upon non-pharmacological approaches and methods. Although evidence is not extensive, some randomised controlled studies have shown beneficial effects for physical exercise alone, combined physical activity with cognitive tasks, and cognitive interventions alone. Barber *et al.* (2012) describe preliminary evidence from randomised controlled trials for physical activity interventions conferring protection from neuronal loss, and preserving neuronal function both through direct effects upon brain regulatory and metabolic mechanisms and through effects upon vascular health.

Law *et al.* (2014) reported a study of 83 Chinese elders with MCI in Hong Kong, comparing a 10-week programme of functional cognitive tasks combined with physical activity (FcTSim) with cognitive training only (computer-based exercises and strategy training). FcTSim incorporated cognitive exercises, specified functional movement practice, simulated functional tasks (such as object placing and collection) and interspersed transfer movements. Subjects were assessed at baseline, immediately after 10 weeks and followed up at six months. The authors found consistently greater intervention effects for the FcTSim group at 10 weeks, persisting at six months, in general cognitive functions, functional status and problem-solving ability. This supports the use of 'real-life' or simulated activities that make both novel and varying cognitive and physical demands upon the person, to improve cognitive function. Underlying mechanisms may be those deriving from physical exercise that support neuronal function and plasticity, combined with those deriving from cognitive challenges that make use of plasticity and support dendritic arborisation and long-term synaptic potentiation.

Rojas *et al.* (2013) undertook a small study randomising 46 older subjects into a control (no treatment) group or an intervention group. The intervention group received a six-month cognitive intervention programme incorporating group activities that provided non-specific social and cognitive stimulation, and training regimes targeted at specific cognitive skills. Like other similar studies, results were mixed, though showing longer term (at one year) differences in some cognitive subtests, and also in conversion rates between the two groups from MCI to dementia (four of the control subjects and one from the intervention group progressed to dementia in the study period). It was, however, a small study. The work by Barnes *et al.* (2004) and Haslam *et al.* (2014) described earlier in Table 11.1 further reinforces the evidence for the value of social group engagement, for both prevention and reduction in rate of cognitive decline.

Although evidence is currently limited, there are indications that interventions involving social engagement, cognitive stimulation and physical activity are not only effective in reducing risk of MCI, but continue to confer benefit for those affected, by slowing deterioration and/or progression to dementia. Hence, for all ages and populations, occupations that incorporate these elements should be encouraged and maintained, linking back to the principles of MECC and to active attention to health promotion in all occupational therapy interventions.

Occupational Therapy – Assessment and Intervention in MCI

There are five reasons, argued above, why occupational therapists should be involved in assessment and intervention in MCI.

1) MCI is prevalent in the older population.
2) It is an indicator for high risk of developing dementia.
3) It negatively impacts performance of IADL.
4) Objective IADL assessment shows potential as a valuable tool for detection and measurement of MCI.
5) MCI appears amenable to occupational interventions to slow progression and maintain function.

Currently there is limited evidence for specific assessment and intervention practices. What there is supports detection through activity-based as well as cognitive assessment, prevention of further decline through health promotion and risk minimisation approaches, and intervention related to specific areas of function, for example:

- the use of objective performance-based measures of ADL, with an emphasis upon IADL
- early engagement to enable people to develop and incorporate preventive and health-maintaining behaviours within daily life, giving attention to psychological, physical and social dimensions
- programmes of cognitive stimulation, social stimulation and physical activity may all confer cognitive benefit.

For assessment, two objective measures of IADL have shown promising results in studies described earlier (Puente *et al.* 2014; Rodakowski *et al.* 2014) – the PASS and the DAFS-R. Both tools include assessment tasks that have a cognitive emphasis, represent higher cognitive demand and are realistic and relevant (including tasks such as medication management). Both have shown an ability to discriminate between task performance by subjects with MCI and normal subjects. Further, they have demonstrated sensitivity equivalent to or greater than standard cognitive tests. For more detailed description of the DAFS-R, see McDougall *et al.* (2010), and for the PASS see Chisholm *et al.* (2014).

For intervention, what evidence there is suggests that programmes of activity should incorporate cognitive challenge (general stimulation and targeted at specific functions), group social interaction and physical activity. Giebel and Challis (2014) reviewed the literature on the relationship between cognitive and ADL deficits in MCI and mild dementia, and interventions to address these. They found that functional interventions generally lacked a theoretical basis, i.e. that activities were not selected for the match between their cognitive demand and the specific cognitive deficits that may underlie performance difficulties, and hence the underlying mechanisms for effectiveness or otherwise of an intervention were difficult to identify. Although the reviewed studies mostly described effective interventions, their heterogeneity, lack of theoretical grounding and generally weak quality ratings made it difficult to draw any firm conclusions. Very few studies have as yet been published that address ADL and IADL interventions specifically.

For specific cognitive deficits, considered elsewhere in this book, there are usually a number of assessment tools, methods and intervention approaches and techniques that can be suggested or recommended, with varying degrees and quality of evidence in support. It may be argued that where specific cognitive functions are affected more than others (for example, memory deficits in amnestic-MCI) then appropriate and focused assessments and interventions will be relevant. In general, considerable further work needs to be done.

The prevalence of MCI, the risk factors for it and its relationship to dementia make occupation-focused assessments and interventions important areas for further research and development.

SUMMARY

1) This chapter has set out the case for a broader consideration of cognitive impairment, in the context of an ageing population and the recognition of major risk factors for chronic ill health and disability in later years.

2) The relationship to dementia and the increasing evidence for its impact upon instrumental activities of daily living make MCI an important condition for occupational therapists to be aware of and understand. The case may be made that they have a substantial role to play in prevention, diagnosis and intervention.

3) The prevalence of chronic ill health conditions in older adults, the economic and social burden created and the suffering experienced by individuals and families as a result demand attention to prevention and promotion of good health across the life-course. Lifestyle factors play a significant role in the genesis of these chronic conditions, including MCI, which requires a major effort from all health professionals, educators and social care workers to fully incorporate health promotion into their work.

4) Although research is relatively recent and sparse, emerging evidence suggests that MCI has greater adverse impacts upon instrumental ADL than previously thought, but also that such activities hold promise for both assessment and intervention.

References

American Psychiatric Association (2013) *Diagnostic and Statistical Manual of Mental Disorders*, 5th edn, American Psychiatric Association, Arlington, Virginia.

Barber, S.E., Clegg, A.P. and Young, J.B. (2012) Is there a role for physical activity in preventing cognitive decline in people with mild cognitive impairment? *Age and Ageing*, **41**, 5–8.

Barnes, L.L., Wilson, R.S. and Evans, D.A. (2004) Social resources and cognitive decline in a population of older African Americans and whites. *Neurology*, **63** (12), 2322–2326.

Barnett, K., Mercer, S.W., Norbury, M., Watt, G., Wyke, S. and Guthrie, B. (2012) Epidemiology of multimorbidity and implications for health care, research, and medical education: a cross-sectional study. *Lancet*, **380**, 37–43.

Bishop, N.A., Lu, T. and Yankner, B.A. (2010) Neural mechanisms of ageing and cognitive decline. *Nature*, **464**, 529–535.

Boyle, P.A., Buchman, A.S., Wilson, R.S., Leurgans, S.E. and Bennett, D.A. (2010) Physical frailty is associated with incident mild cognitive impairment in community-based older persons. *Journal of the American Psychiatric Society*, **58**, 248–255.

Brinke, ten, L.F., Bolandzadeh, N., Nagamatsu, L.S. *et al.* (2015) Aerobic exercise increases hippocampal volume in older women with probable mild cognitive impairment: a 6-month randomised controlled trial. *British Journal of Sports Medicine*, **49**, 248–254.

Buchman, A.S., Boyle, P.A., Wilson, R.S., Tang, Y. and Bennett, D.A. (2007) Frailty is associated with incident Alzheimer's disease and cognitive decline in the elderly. *Psychosomatic Medicine*, **69**, 483–489.

Butler, R.N., Forette, F. and Greengross, S. (2004) Maintaining cognitive health in an ageing society. *Journal of the Royal Society for the Promotion of Health*, **124** (3), 119–121.

Chisholm, D., Toto, P., Raina, K., Holm, M. and Rogers, J. (2014) Evaluating capacity to live independently and safely in the community: Performance Assessment of Self-care Skills. *British Journal of Occupational Therapy*, **77** (2), 59–63.

Cholerton, B., Baker, L.D. and Craft, S. (2011) Review article: insulin resistance and pathological brain ageing. *Diabetic Medicine*, **28** (12), 1463–1475.

Clegg, A., Young, J., Iliffe, S., Rikkert, M.O. and Rockwood, K. (2013) Frailty in elderly people. *Lancet*, **381**, 752–762.

Colcombe, S. and Kramer, A.F. (2003) Fitness effects on the cognitive function of older adults: a meta-analytic study. *Psychological Science*, **14** (2), 125–130.

Colcombe, S.J., Erickson, K.I., Scalf, P.E. *et al.* (2006) Aerobic exercise training increases brain volume in aging humans. *Journal of Gerontology*, **61A** (11), 1166–1170.

Department of Health (2011) *Start Active, Stay Active: A Report on Physical Activity from the Four Home Countries' Chief Medical Officers*. Department of Health, London.

De Vriendt, P., Gorus, E., Cornelis, E. *et al.* (2013) The advanced activities of daily living: a tool allowing the evaluation of subtle functional decline in mild cognitive impairment. *Journal of Nutrition, Health and Aging*, **17** (1), 64–71.

East Midlands Health Trainer Hub (undated) *An Implementation Guide and Toolkit for Making Every Contact Count*. Trent Publications. Available at: www.makingeverycontactcount.co.uk/MECC%20In%20Action/Implementing%20 MECC/Toolkit.html (accessed 27 September 2016).

Giebel, C. and Challis, D. (2014) Translating cognitive and everyday activity deficits into cognitive interventions in mild dementia and mild cognitive impairment. *International Journal of Geriatric Psychiatry*, **30**, 21–31.

Haslam, C., Cruwys, T. and Haslam, S.A. (2014) 'The we's have it': evidence for the distinctive benefits of group engagement in enhancing cognitive health in aging. *Social Science and Medicine*, **120**, 57–66.

Hotting, K. and Roder, B. (2013) Beneficial effects of physical exercise on neuroplasticity and cognition. *Neuroscience and Behavioural Reviews*, **37**, 2243–2257.

Kanoski, S.E. and Davidson, T.L. (2011) Western diet consumption and cognitive impairment: links to hippocampal dysfunction and obesity. *Physiology and Behaviour*, **103**, 59–68.

King's Fund (2015) Life expectancy. Available at: www.kingsfund.org.uk/time-to-think-differently/trends/demography/life-expectancy (accessed 27 September 2016).

Kuh, D. (2007) A life course approach to healthy aging, frailty, and capability. *Journal of Gerontology*, **62A** (7), 717–721.

Law, L.F.L., Barnett, F., Yau, M.K. and Gray, M.A. (2014) Effects of functional tasks exercise on older adults with cognitive impairment at risk of Alzheimer's disease: a randomised controlled trial. *Age and Ageing*, **43**, 813–820.

McDougall, G.J., Becker, H., Vaughan P.W., Acee, T.W. and Delville, C.L. (2010) The Revised Direct Assessment of Functional status for Independent Older adults. *Gerontologist*, **50** (3), 363–370.

NHS Future Forum (2012) *The NHS's Role in the Public's Health: A Report from the NHS Future Forum*. NHS Future Forum. Available at: www.gov.uk/government/publications/nhs-future-forum-recommendations-to-government-second-phase (accessed 30 September 2016).

Park S.K., Richardson, C.R., Holleman, R.G. and Larson, J.L. (2013) Frailty in people with COPD, using the National Health and Nutrition Evaluation Survey dataset (2003–2006). *Heart and Lung*, **42**, 163–170.

Partridge, J.S.L., Dhesi, J.K., Cross, J.D. *et al.* (2014) The prevalence and impact of undiagnosed cognitive impairment in older vascular surgical patients. *Journal of Vascular Surgery*, **60** (4), 1002–1011.

Percival, J. (2014) Promoting health: making every contact count. *Nursing Standard*, **28** (29), 37–41.

Petersen, R.C., Caracciolo, B., Brayne, S., Gauthier, S., Jelic, V. and Fratiglioni, L. (2014) Mild cognitive impairment: a concept in evolution. *Journal of Internal Medicine*, **275**, 214–228.

Prince, M., Knapp, M., Guerchet, M. *et al.* (2014) *Dementia UK Update*. Alzheimer's Society, Cardiff.

Puente, A.N., Terry, D.P., Faraco, C.C., Brown, C.L. and Miller, L.S. (2014) Functional impairment in mild cognitive impairment evidenced using performance-based measurement. *Journal of Geriatric Psychiatry and Neurology*, **27** (4), 253–258.

Reppermund, S., Brodaty, H., Crawford, J.D. *et al.* (2013) Impairment in instrumental activities of daily living with high cognitive demand is an early marker of mild cognitive impairment: the Sydney Memory and Ageing Study. *Psychological Medicine*, **43**, 2437–2445.

Rodakowski, J., Skidmore, E.R., Reynolds, C.F. *et al.* (2014) Can performance on daily activities discriminate between older adults with normal cognitive function and those with mild cognitive impairment? *Journal of the American Geriatrics Society*, **62**, 1347–1352.

Rojas, G.J., Villar, V., Iturry, M. *et al.* (2013) Efficacy of a cognitive intervention program in patients with mild cognitive impairment. *International Psychogeriatrics*, **25** (5), 825–831.

Sachdev, P.S., Lipnicki, D.M., Crawford, J. *et al.* for the Memory and Ageing Study Team (2012) Risk profiles of subtypes of mild cognitive impairment: the Sydney Memory and Ageing Study. *Journal of the American Geriatrics Society*, **60**, 24–33.

Sachs-Ericsson, N. and Blazer, D.G. (2015) The new DSM-5 diagnosis of mild neurocognitive disorder and its relation to research in mild cognitive impairment. *Aging and Mental Health*, **19** (1), 2–12.

Singh, B., Parsaik, A.K., Mielke, M.M. *et al.* (2013) Chronic obstructive pulmonary disease and association with mild cognitive impairment: the Mayo Clinic study of aging. *Mayo Clinic Proceedings*, **88** (11), 1222–1230.

Tournoy, J., Lee, D.M., Pendleton, N. *et al.* for the EMAS Study Group (2010) Association of cognitive performance with the metabolic syndrome and with glycaemia in middle-aged and older European men: the European Male Ageing Study. *Diabetes/Metabolism Research and Reviews*, **26**, 668–676.

Wendell, C.R., Zonderman, A.B., Metter, E.J., Najjar, S.S. and Waldstein, S.R. (2009) Carotid intimal medial thickness predicts cognitive decline among adults without clinical vascular disease. *Stroke*, **40** (10), 3180–3185.

Wendell, C.R., Gunstad, J., Waldstein, S.R., Wright, J.G., Ferrucci, L. AND Zonderman, A.B. (2014) Cardiorespiratory fitness and accelerated cognitive decline with aging. *Journals of Gerontology A: Biological Sciences and Medical Sciences*, **69** (4), 455–462.

Wennberg, A.M.V., Gottesman, R.F., Kaufmann, C.N. *et al.* (2014) Diabetes and cognitive outcomes in a nationally representative sample: the National Health and Aging Trends Study. *International Psychogeriatrics*, **26** (10), 1729–1735.

Wilson, V.K., Houston, D.K., Kilpatrick, L. *et al.* (2014) Relationship between 25-hydroxyvitamin D and cognitive function in older adults: the Health, Aging and Body Composition Study. *Journal of the American Geriatrics Society*, **62**, 636–641.

Yates, K.F., Sweat, V., Yau, P.L., Turchiano, M.M. and Convit, A. (2012) Impact of metabolic syndrome on cognition and brain: a selected review of the literature. *Arteriosclerosis Thrombosis and Vascular Biology*, **32** (9), 2060–2067.

Index

Note: Where index items are located within tables or figures, page numbers in **bold** denote tables, and numbers in *italics* denote figures

Neuropsychology for Occupational Therapists: Cognition in Occupational Performance, Fourth Edition.
Edited by Linda Maskill and Stephanie Tempest.
© 2017 John Wiley & Sons Ltd. Published 2017 by John Wiley & Sons Ltd.
Companion Website: www.wiley.com/go/maskill/neuropsychologyOT

Made in the USA
Columbia, SC
10 July 2021

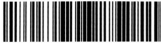